Understanding Everyday Experience
Series Editor: Laurie Taylor

For Anna, Melanie and Holly

STEVI JACKSON

Childhood and Sexuality

Basil Blackwell · Oxford

First published 1982
Basil Blackwell Publisher Limited
108 Cowley Road, Oxford OX4 1JF, England

British Library Cataloguing in Publication Data

Jackson Stevi
    Childhood and sexuality. — (Understanding everyday
    experience)
    1. Children—Sexual behavior
    I. Title   II. Series
    306.7   HQ784.S45

    ISBN 0-631-12871-9
    ISBN 0-631-12949-9 Pbk

Typesetting by Cambrian Typesetters
Farnborough, Hants
Printed in Great Britain by The Camelot Press, Southampton

Contents

Acknowledgements

I would like to thank all the friends and colleagues who have, in various ways, contributed to this book. Those who have offered ideas, criticism and encouragement include Deirdre Beddoe, Peter Brunsdon, Mary Dalton, Eva Eberhardt, Frances Jackson, Chris Jones, Andy Moye, Rose Pearson, Pete Rushton, Laurie Taylor, Jean Thirtle and Glyn Watson. I also owe an enormous debt to the women's movement, without which many of the issues raised in these pages would never have surfaced and which has been for me a constant source of inspiration.

I would like to thank Hamish Hamilton Ltd for permission to quote from L.P Hartley's *The Go-Between* and the estate of Carson McCullers for permission to quote from *The Member of the Wedding*.

Preface

Stevi Jackson's original title for this book was *Children and Sex*. It was certainly the simplest phrase to cover her investigation into our attitudes towards the subject and her discussion of how such attitudes might affect the lives of our own children.

But it worried the publishers a little, and was thought likely to worry potential readers even more. The mere combination of the words seemed to raise disturbing spectres: was this a pornographic text, a celebration of paedophilia, a plea for infantile promiscuity?

Perhaps she should have expected such a reaction. For, as she says in her opening chapter: 'To write about children and sex is to bring together two sets of issues that are highly emotive, that readily provoke moral outrage and righteous indignation. Virtually everyone has firm opinions on these matters, and some have unshakeable convictions.' In the face of such potential reactions, she settled — after some argument — for the safer academic title which the book now enjoys.

But this has been the only concession. Stevi Jackson has elsewhere refused to abandon her intention to write with considerable candour about matters which are usually either left unsaid, or buried beneath a mass of hypocrisies and euphemisms. For although we may choose to describe our present society as relatively libertarian, or even sexually permissive, as she vividly shows there is little in our attitudes towards children and sex to suggest that we have done anything to confront quite fundamental fears and anxieties.

It may seem odd to include a book on this subject in a series entitled *Understanding Everyday Experience*. But as Ms Jackson makes plain, it is our refusal to acknowledge the everyday, even the mundane, character of the experiences she describes that has led them to become the preserve of the expert: the psychiatrist, the sex educator, the counsellor.

This means that the present volume sits easily alongside the earlier books in the series, which have been devoted to such everyday but problematic matters as ageing and disability. And, like those other books, its success may be measured by the extent to which it persuades the reader, whether parent, teacher or young person, that here is an area far too important to be handed over to the specialist.

It may be the case, as Stevi Jackson argues, that the idea of 'true sexual freedom' for children can, as long as we live in our present society, only be a utopian desire. But this does not provide an excuse for inaction. In her words, 'if we do not try we are colluding in the perpetuation of sexual coercion and exploitation, of sexual guilt, of the oppression of women and children.'

Laurie Taylor

1

Breaking Taboos

Any statement about children and sex is almost guaranteed to be controversial: a book on the subject cannot avoid offending some of its readers. To write about children and sex is to bring together two sets of issues that are highly emotive, that readily provoke moral outrage and righteous indignation. Virtually everyone has firm opinions on these matters, and some have unshakeable convictions.

In modern Western societies children are set apart from the rest of the population, regarded as a special category of people with their own needs. We have particular obligations towards them: we are expected to protect and take care of them, to put their interests before our own. Any event or circumstance that affects them, especially if it is seen as placing them 'at risk', easily becomes a public issue. In a sense children are ideal victims, creatures peculiarly deserving of our sympathy, so that any real or imaginary threat to them can be used to manipulate public opinion. Charities soliciting funds, politicians seeking votes and advertisers selling soup and soap powder all know that if they focus their campaigns on children they are more likely to get the response they want. Most of us can be counted on to react emotionally to situations where children are threatened in some way, whether by natural disasters, inadequate educational facilities or even our failure to buy them the right brand of baked beans. The fate of children occupies a special place in the popular imagination.

Sexuality is also a provocative topic, a fit subject for public scandals and moral crusades. Whenever such issues as homosexuality, pornography or prostitution are raised, or when the unconventional behavior of a group of people or the indiscretions of a celebrity are made public, intense interest is aroused. Banner headlines appear in the press, politicians make statements, indignant letters are written to radio stations and newspapers. As public debate unfolds, predictable battle lines are drawn between liberal proponents of sexual 'freedom' and conservative campaigners against sexual 'permissiveness'. On both sides of the moral barricades sexuality is singled out as a special area of life, as sacred or taboo, as elevating or degrading. Of course, there is a wide spectrum of opinion, but there are extremists on both sides. Some see sexual repression as the root of all modern evil and freedom of sexual expression as the path to salvation. Other people fear that civilization is about to be submerged altogether under a rising tide of libidinous licence. Only rarely is sexuality accepted as a routine part of everyday life, as something that can be discussed with ease; indeed, whether it should be talked about at all is still a contentious issue.

If we regard children as a special category of people and sexuality as a special area of life, then any meeting between the two is likely to be explosive. Not only are both subjects controversial in their own right, but bringing them together breaks a particularly powerful social taboo: that children and sex should be kept apart.

Since Freud first suggested that children are sexual the idea has gradually, but only grudgingly, become accepted. Children are still not generally treated as sexual beings and the possibility that they might be makes many of us feel uneasy. Sexuality remains an aspect of life that we tend to conceal from them and regard as dangerous to them. Recently I heard a letter read on the radio in which the correspondent deplored the increase in sexual information available to young people today. In her youth, she said, children had grown up much happier without such knowledge, their innocence untarnished, and they did not learn about the 'seamy side' of life until they married. Although such views may seem old-fashioned, many still hold them. I suspect, too, that many people who would challenge these attitudes and assert that there is nothing sordid about sex would still feel it inappropriate for younger children to know about sex. Even people whose outlooks are radical or libertarian sometimes claim that young children cannot understand sex and will only be confused and frightened by it.

Many rules and conventions exist to define sex as the preserve of adults: age of consent laws, selective censorship practices, the labelling of erotic books as 'adult literature' and so on. These are the outward signs of the taboo surrounding children and sex, and even to question them is to invite a hostile response. A heated debate surrounds any issue that links children and sex, whether child pornography, sex education or children's exposure to sexual scenes on television. A particularly contentious question is the degree of access children should have to sexual information and experience, and when and how it should be gained. Sex education is seen by some people as a means of dispelling ignorance and by others as despoiling innocence. Some say it should enable young people to enjoy sex without guilt; others think it should warn young people of the dangers of sexual contact until such time as religious rites or legal contracts have made it 'safe'.

The issues at stake are often not as clear-cut as they might appear. Their complexity is commonly concealed behind predictable moral stances. We often use terms like 'promiscuity' and 'permissiveness', 'repression' and 'freedom' without making it at all clear what we mean by them. Everyone claims to have the interests of children at heart, but it sometimes happens that these interests are threatened by our attitudes and policies. Take, for example, the thorny issue of age of consent laws, which are supposed to protect the young from sexual exploitation. Because of them, girls may find it difficult to obtain reliable forms of contraception and thus risk unwanted pregnancy. Since the double standard of sexual morality is built into these laws, they might also find themselves labelled as 'sexual delinquents'; there are many girls in Britain and the United States who have been confined to institutions for young offenders for the sole crime of 'promiscuity'. Problems like this lead some people to argue that these laws are repressive and unjust and should be abolished. Yet it might also be argued that repealing them, or lowering their age limits, would equally restrict freedom in a society where sexual coercion and exploitation is commonplace. The National Council for Civil Liberties in Britain claims that the existing laws on sexual assault and rape would prevent this happening, but the failure of these laws to protect adult women gives no cause for optimism. There is, then, no easy means

4

of resolving this issue; the same is true of many others concerning children and sex.

The debates surrounding such questions cannot be ignored, and I hope this book will add to them. I will no doubt stray into areas some people would wish untouched, and challenge values some would prefer to leave unquestioned. My aim is to examine our attitudes to children and sex; to explore the assumptions that underlie the competing moral positions on the subject; and to consider what effects our attitudes have on our own and others' children as they learn about sexuality and come to terms with their own sexual experience.

In doing this I will raise a number of questions about aspects of life we usually take for granted. Do we learn how to be sexual or is sexuality wholly inborn? Is childhood a natural state or a social status? How and why do adults conceal sex from children, and what are the consequences? Are children sexual beings and, if so, in what sense? How do most children actually acquire sexual information, and what do they make of it? Is it possible or desirable to make changes in the ways we deal with children and sex? Some of these questions are more familiar than others, but I hope that asking them will give us the chance to pause and think about our everyday behaviour. In our relationships with children we sometimes feel the need to examine our own motives and intentions or to explain them to others, but most of the time we are not so self-conscious. Even when we do form explanations we often base them on attitudes and ideas that are seldom or never questioned. I plan to question them here.

This book is an attempt to break the silence that surrounds the subject of children and sex, to explore hidden fears and anxieties, to expose unspoken assumptions. This is a subject that affects all of us at some time in our lives and I would like to think that everyone will find something of interest in what I have to say. I hope that in particular parents, teachers and all those involved in caring for children will think it useful to consider the issues I raise. Nor would it do any harm for young people themselves to read what follows.

2

It's Only Natural . . .
Or Is It?

Among the many concepts we use to make sense of everyday experience are ideas about 'human nature', about what counts as 'natural' or 'unnatural'. In judging people or situations by this particular yardstick we seem to be appealing to facts, but we are also making moral judgements. To call something 'natural' generally implies that it is good and acceptable, or at least excusable; to label something 'unnatural' is to damn it as indefensible.

Nowhere are ideas about naturalness more entrenched than in attitudes to sexuality. The very phrase 'unnatural acts' conjures up images of bizarre and distasteful sexual practices. The more usual forms of sexual behaviour in our society, on the other hand, are often assumed to be natural, products of inbuilt needs and drives rather than expressions of custom and convention. According to this view the influence of society is only slight, operating through moral values that repress our basic drives or channel them in acceptable directions.

Naturalness is thus a standard usually invoked to defend particular values or behaviour. For example, it has become fashionable to argue that sex, being 'natural', is therefore wholesome and good, so that puritanical attitudes are at best inappropriate and at worst destructively repressive. The equation between naturalness and goodness, however, does not always hold where sexuality is concerned. An older tradition regards nature as a less benign influence, one which must be conquered if civilized human society is to prosper. Sexuality may be thought of as particularly threatening, representing the baser aspects of human nature, our animal side, a dangerous force kept in check only by a thin veneer of civilization. The moral concern that surrounds the alleged permissiveness of young people, pornography, marital breakdown and so on, frequently prompts statements that society will collapse if this powerful urge is allowed to get out of hand. It is interesting that opposing viewpoints are based on the same assumption: that sexual behaviour is natural. There are differences of opinion about which forms of sexual activity count as natural, and about whether nature should be given free reign, but the idea that there is a basic human sexual nature is rarely challenged.

Ideas about naturalness will obviously have an impact on our attitudes to children and sex and affect the ways we see and judge children's emerging sexuality. Is it natural or unnatural for children to be aware of sexuality? What is the natural pace of sexual development? Should we teach children the value of self-control, or allow them 'free' expression of their sexuality? As a first step towards clarifying these issues, we need to examine the idea of naturalness around which they revolve.

It is not difficult to understand why sex is so likely to be seen as something determined by biology. Our ideas of sexual attractiveness and competence are linked to physical maturity, and after all, sexuality is part of a basic biological process — reproduction. Culture, however, plays a much larger part in moulding our sexuality than we usually realize. Nature has endowed us with certain sexual capacities, but it does not dictate how we express them. We may at times feel we are acting out compelling desires through our sexual relationships, but this does not mean that the desires or the behaviour they prompt are purely instinctual.

The belief that human sexuality is governed by instincts is usually backed up by two kinds of pseudo-scientific theory. The first is that our sexual behaviour is governed by mysterious substances called hormones. The second assumes that, since sex is an activity basic to all animal life, its human form must follow patterns similar to those of other species, or alternatively must represent evolutionary adaptations vital to the survival of our own.

The effects of hormones on sexual feelings and actions are frequently over-estimated. Hormones are a vital part of our body chemistry; we manufacture several and they perform a variety of functions. However, their impact on the way we feel and act is by no means direct. Injecting rats with a particular hormone may produce predictable results, but the same is not true for people. We do not simply react to a particular physical stimulus; we endow our actions with meaning and respond to other influences at the same time. For example, if adrenalin is administered to human subjects they can experience a range of emotions including fear, anger and euphoria, depending on their situation and the behaviour of others. The effects of the hormone are thus modified by social factors.

9

It is the androgens, or 'male' hormones, that endow both women and men with the capacity for sexual arousal. However, despite the fact that sexual arousal is a physiological state and can be measured scientifically, it is not simply the product of internal chemical reactions. If a female rat is injected with androgens she becomes more sexually aggressive. A woman's response will vary, depending upon her feelings about what is happening and how she can express them. Until she acknowledges that she is sexually aroused it is doubtful that she will even experience coherent desires or fantasies. Whether or not she acts on her feelings may depend on a range of external circumstances, as will the way she acts — perhaps a brisk walk, solitary masturbation or love-making with a partner.

Evidence from studies of women with abnormally high androgen levels suggests that although hormones may affect the ease with which we become sexually aroused, they have no apparent impact on any other aspect of our sexuality. These women may become aroused exceptionally easily, but their sexual desires and fantasies are similar to those of 'normal' women.

Although hormones are often talked about as if they careered through our bodies determining our actions in mysterious and uncontrollable ways, their effects on our sexual lives are actually very limited. Human sexuality is not just a matter of instinctual urges; it includes all kinds of behaviour and relationships that cannot be explained merely by what we know about the chemicals in the body.

Another way of arguing that sexual behaviour is natural is to stress its 'animal' characteristics. This version of the argument has been backed by the work of writers such as Desmond Morris, Robert Ardrey, and Lionel Tiger and Robin Fox, who all attempt to demonstrate continuities between human and animal behaviour. Judging from the commercial success of such books as *The Naked Ape, African Genesis* and *The Imperial Animal*, this argument has great popular appeal, suggesting that for some reason many people enjoy being told that they behave like baboons.

The fallacy of deducing what is natural for humans from observing other species should be obvious: we are capable of a far wider and more complex range of behaviour than any other animal. As the psychologist Naomi Weisstein has pointed out, one logical conclusion of the argument would be that 'it is quite useless to teach human infants to speak since it has been tried with chimpanzees and does not work.'

Most of those who draw parallels between human and animal behaviour do recognize, of course, that people are in some sense more sophisticated, but they insist that this sophistication is just a development of characteristics we share with other species, especially the primates. In the search for qualities that we share with animals, however, our ideas of our own natures are likely to intervene and determine which features we select as held in common and therefore natural. So it is not surprising that authors writing in this vein should disagree on some fundamental aspects of human sexuality, even though they draw on similar kinds of evidence, For example, Desmond Morris asserts that we are naturally a monogamous species while Tiger and Fox insist that we are polygynous. They all agree that the male is the natural aggressor in heterosexual encounters, while Robert Ardrey claims that this view originates in modern moral values and that, in fact, the female is naturally the initiator and aggressor in sex. It seems that when they examined

11

the evidence, these writers simply found what they were looking for. Indeed, it is possible to 'prove' that almost any human activity is natural simply by selecting and interpreting information about animal behaviour to suit one's own cherished beliefs.

One of the earliest and most popular books of this kind, and one which has much to say about sexuality, is Desmond Morris's *The Naked Ape*. Here it is argued that the forms of sexual behaviour typical of Americans and Europeans are part of a biological pattern. According to Morris, *Homo sapiens* is 'the sexiest primate alive' because our capacity for arousal is not tied to female fertility cycles. It is this basic fact, to which Morris attaches a great deal of importance, that should warn us against viewing human sexuality as biologically determined, for it implies that our sexual feelings are *not* triggered by hormones, that we respond to more subtle forms of stimulation, and that influences other than biological ones might affect our arousal. Undeterred by these matters, however, Morris continues to look to biology to explain what turns us on, and argues that many specifically human anatomical features, such as the shape of our lips and the female breast, have developed purely as sexual signalling devices. Having developed these characteristics in order to 'make sex sexier' and thus cement the bond between couples, as he argues, we have then developed strategies (apparently just as 'natural') to make sure we don't accidentally attract someone other than our partner.

The fallacy of arguing that we respond directly to certain predetermined stimuli is easily demonstrated if we call on common sense and personal experience. Consider the act of touching a woman's genitals. In Morris's terms this is a sexual act and ought to produce

12

instant arousal. This may be true if the person is the woman's lover, but if she or he is a doctor conducting a gynaecological examination the situation will not be seen as sexual and is unlikely to be experienced as erotic. Even if a woman's genitals are caressed with obvious sexual intent, it will not necessarily arouse her if she is not feeling sexually inclined at that moment or is not attracted to the person concerned.

Our biological make-up has indeed, as Morris points out, provided us with a complex range of signalling devices — language, gestures, facial expressions — that can be used to ease communication in many situations, including sexual ones. But these signals are not erotic by themselves; they need to be interpreted as such before anything sexual is likely to occur. In the early stages of a sexual encounter or relationship in our culture it is not considered appropriate to state our intentions openly. Instead we proceed by gesture and innuendo, cues which have to be interpreted correctly before we obtain a sexual response. If these signals were part of our biological make-up interpretation would not be necessary and they would never be ambiguous — which they frequently are. It is common to experience a period of uncertainty, especially at the beginning of sexual negotiations, when we are unsure whether the signals we are receiving are sexual or whether the other person is aware of what we are signalling.

Not only are sexual signals open to misinterpretation, but our ability to become aroused may be entirely unrelated to them. Because we have imagination, we may become aroused by some activity or characteristic of someone we desire that at the time has nothing to do with sex. It has been observed, for example, that people often watch the hands of someone they are attracted to. In Marilyn French's novel *The Women's Room*, the exuberant Val counts it as part of the process of becoming infatuated: 'You can't look at his hands without imagining them on your body. Looking at his hands becomes a forbidden act, an act of lasciviousness.' It is not the hands themselves that are erotic, nor what they are doing, but the imagining of what they *could* do.

Morris's depiction of sexual arousal as a direct response to given stimuli, then, seems not to reflect experience. Neither do the explanations he offers for other aspects of sexual normality.

There are other and less subjective ways of countering the claim that conventional patterns of sexual behaviour are natural, in particular by looking at the anthropological evidence. If these patterns were natural to our species they would have been adopted by all peoples at all times, which is clearly not so. Biological determinists prefer to ignore these facts. Morris asserts that the practices of other societies can be ignored since they 'no longer represent the mainstream of evolution'. But the inhabitants of the Western world have not actually evolved biologically beyond other peoples: we are merely culturally different. Lionel Tiger and Robin Fox in *The Imperial Animal* offer a more sophisticated approach. They argue that all varieties of human culture are merely variations on a few biologically fixed themes. This, too, is misleading. The example offered by Tiger and Fox is that courtship occurs in all societies. Given that sexual relationships are universal, this merely states the obvious: that means must be found for communicating sexual intentions and for translating them into action. Beyond this, we learn little about the reality of people's lives. If we are to arrive at a

14

fuller understanding of sexuality, or of any other aspect of human activity, we can no more afford to rely on such broad generalizations than we can afford to define our customs as 'natural' and dismiss all others as the exotic predilections of primitive peoples.

Human sexuality certainly does have a biological basis, in that nature has endowed us with a certain sexual potential, but this does not make it biologically *determined* or any more 'natural' than other aspects of human behaviour. Eating is biologically necessary, but we do not see our eating habits as ordained by nature: it would be absurd for an Italian to maintain that all human beings are genetically programmed to enjoy the taste of pasta, or for a Chinese to claim that using chopsticks is a natural aptitude. There are as many cultural variations in sexual practices and preferences as there are in eating habits; the biological raw material of human sexuality may be moulded into a range of distinctive forms. Around the basic facts of anatomy, physiology and physical development are woven complex cultural webs to produce a whole spectrum of behaviour and relationships that testifies to the malleability of our sexual nature. No doubt members of every society assume that their particular form of sexuality is natural, but other people's ideas of what is natural may be very different from our own.

Culture's most obvious influence on sexuality, one we are all aware of at some time, is in the creation of moral boundaries defining the limits of acceptable sexual behaviour. All societies have rules governing who may enter into sexual relations with whom, how, when and in what context, but the content of these rules, the degree to which they restrict the individual and the extent to which they are obeyed vary greatly.

15

Although we may be aware of the moral standards that impinge upon us, we are usually far less conscious of the many other, more fundamental, ways in which culture shapes our sexuality. Almost every aspect of sexual life involves different patterns of behaviour in different cultures. In some societies sex is primarily experienced as a routine, though pleasureable, part of everyday existence; in others it is commonly thought to be potentially dangerous and polluting and is the source of much anxiety. Sexual intercourse may be regarded primarily as a gesture of affection or as the culmination of violent passion. There are societies where sexual encounters involve nothing more than brief acts of intercourse, others where more prolonged and elaborate forms of eroticism are usual. Some peoples insist that women are the sexual aggressors and are more highly sexed than men, while elsewhere, as in our own society, the opposite view is held. Within some cultures a great deal of emphasis is placed on differences between female and male sexuality; in others no distinctions are made.

There is great diversity too, in what people experience as erotic. A gesture implying sexual interest or invitation in one society may not carry this message elsewhere, and an activity which contributes to arousal among some peoples might be thought repugnant or merely amusing by others. We may think that it is 'only natural' that certain things 'turn us on', but we would usually be wrong.

A well-documented illustration is the kiss. Kissing is considered so natural in Western societies that it is tempting to say that it is what lips are for — indeed, Desmond Morris claims that this is precisely why they evolved as a distinctive human feature. The kiss is an essential element in our sexual repertoire, the subject of much romantic and erotic literature; a sexual encounter in which it played no part would seem oddly cold and mechanical. It serves as a boundary, defining the beginning and end of a sexual encounter and featuring prominently in lovers' meetings and partings. It has a symbolic significance, especially in the early stages of a relationship, indicating when it starts to become sexual. It is partly for this reason that we find it erotically stimulating — it both confirms a mutual attraction and promises more to come. But a kiss is also an end in itself, something simultaneously arousing and satisfying. It is extremely versatile too, capable of expressing a range of emotions from affection and tenderness to passionate desire.

Given all this, kissing seems indispensable; yet on a world scale it is a minority activity — most cultures have managed without it. Those Westerners who first observed its absence in Africa, the Far East and the Pacific were apt to consider this a deplorable deficiency. Winwoode Reade, an Englishman travelling in West Africa in the nineteenth century, took a charitable view, urging the readers of his *Savage Africa* not to 'despise the poor untutored African, or judge him too severely on account of an ignorance for which he is not to blame'. Africans were, he considered, to be pitied for their failure to discover this 'civilized method of endearment'.

Observers like Reade, imbued with the confident ethnocentrism of their age, could not help but conclude that other societies were missing out, that it was up to us, the 'superior' race, to teach them the errors of their ways. Yet other peoples' reactions to the Western custom of kissing were often far from enthusiastic; the practice was hardly welcomed as a wonderful erotic delight. When Reade himself first attempted to kiss an African woman she ran away, terrified — her only sources of comparison being snakes' habit of moistening their victims before eating them, and human cannibalism. Once convinced that she was not about to become Reade's dinner, she apparently consented to let him kiss her, but we are not told whether she enjoyed the experience. There is plenty of evidence from elsewhere that would suggest not. Although we have since been more successful in exporting this and other aspects of our culture, members of different societies initially found it either disgusting, as did the Chinese, or just boring or amusing. The anthropologist Malinowski tells how the Trobriand Islanders, having learnt of the white man's penchant for kissing, found it hilarious. They could not imagine how anyone could possibly derive sensual pleasure from so uninspiring an activity. Their reaction was similar to our feelings about the Maori practice of nose-rubbing and the Trobrianders' own custom of biting out each others' eyelashes. Anyone who has tried these techniques will probably not have found them quite as erotic as do the peoples who originated them.

This example suggested that when we think we are simply 'doing what comes naturally' our sense of naturalness derives not from biological facts but from socially contructed definitions of what is sexual. We may 'naturally' have the potential to be aroused by a kiss, but we are similarly capable of being turned on by nose-rubbing or eyelash-biting: if we are not, it is because we have not learnt to consider these activities as aspects of lovemaking. Our erotic sense is not in-born but created through learning to be sexual in a particular society.

It is not surprising then, that almost everything that happens in the course of sexual encounters varies from culture to culture: ways of negotiating sexual relationships, the degree and techniques of foreplay, sexual positions. What passes as sexual competence in one society may even indicate ineptitude in the next: the Trobriand Islands not only found kissing unsatisfying, but considered white men to be incompetent in all sexual techniques.

Even the most intensely sexual of all experiences, the orgasm, is influenced by culture. This is particularly so in the female orgasm, where clearly there is a combination of anatomical and cultural factors at work. The Western woman is not alone in experiencing difficulties in obtaining full sexual satisfaction, but her problems are not the direct result of her biology. In societies where women are expected to be sexually passive, where sex is defined as a male pleasure but a female duty and where non-copulatory sexual activity is at a minimum, women rarely, if ever, achieve orgasm: it is made both physically and psychologically impossible for them. But where women are active rather than passive in sexual encounters, where their right to pleasure is well established, and where sex is not confined to intercourse, no such problems exist. Aboriginal women in north-west Australia sing songs that glorify the role of the clitoris in lovemaking, while in our society it is possible for girls to grow up without even knowing that they have one, and if anyone were enterprising enough to record a song about it, it would no doubt be judged obscene.

Male orgasm, on the other hand, seems much less of a problem, more of an automatic reflex. Since sex in all cultures involves stimulation of the penis, and since any society whose men were physically incapable of orgasm would soon become extinct, this is not surprising. Yet there is one society on record — the Arapesh of New Guinea — where neither male nor female orgasm is recognized. Arapesh men experience ejaculation purely as a loss of erection. The triumph of culture over nature is here complete, for although orgasm occurs physically, it has no erotic significance. The Arapesh do not share our goal-oriented, orgasm-as-finale notion of sexuality but evaluate it in terms of mutual ease and comfort, as a gesture of deep and committed affection rather than as a form of physical gratification.

This inability on the part of men to identify orgasm as a distinct experience may seem startling; it intrigued me enough to make me ask some of my male friends about how far they regard ejaculation and orgasm as the same thing. Most told me that on occasions their ejaculations did not feel very orgasmic, that they did not always experience it as the climax of lovemaking and that it could be empty of meaning and almost devoid of sensation. If men in our society can sometimes feel like this, it seems less surprising that people who are not brought up to see sex as a means of physical gratification do not attach any particular significance to the physical sensations of orgasm.

It seems, then, that the experience of sex is rather more than a cumulation of physical stimuli and sensations — that what makes these things erotic is the meaning given to them. This applies not only to what arouses and satisfies us, but also to the ways in which we identify and experience sexual desire. In responding to this desire we are not acting out inner instincts, but expressing culturally acquired desires through socially acceptable channels.

Given that culture, not nature, shapes the form of

our sexuality, it is clear that most of our sexual behaviour is learnt. This is why childhood is so important, for what we learn in these early years has far more effect on our sexuality than any instinctual urges. We can only understand how we express our sexuality by examining how it develops in childhood and adolescence. In considering how children learn about sex, on the other hand, we must keep in mind the kind of adult sexuality they are learning about. In order to make sense of issues concerning children and sex we should dispense with notions of naturalness.

As sexuality is shaped by culture, its present manifestations can be neither natural nor unnatural. The implications that follow may make many people reluctant to relinquish the notion of naturalness. It means that there are no absolute standards: nature can no longer be the arbiter of our moral disputes. Without nature to lean on, morality has to be based on other criteria, and it is no longer possible to disguise judgements of value as statements of fact.

3

The Nature of Childhood

Having examined the ways in which human sexuality is shaped by society and culture, I will now turn to the other side of the question: the nature of childhood. Just as sex is not merely a product of natural impulses, so childhood is not merely a natural state, for as well as being a stage of physical development it is also a social institution. It has not been defined and experienced in the same way in all societies and at all times. The form childhood takes is shaped by many other aspects of social life such as the means of subsistence available in a particular society, the organization of work and leisure and the typical patterns of family relationships. The place children occupy in a society, the lives they lead, their relationships with adults and adult attitudes toward them are, therefore, part of a much broader social and cultural picture. Our feelings about children and sex are not a natural response to people of a particular age but result from the way childhood is defined within our society.

In modern Western societies children live in a social world separate from that inhabited by adults. Although it is said that we are living in a child-centred society, and the belief that children should be 'seen and not heard' has been eroded, children are excluded by law or convention from many aspects of adult social life, so that there are many places where they are in fact neither seen nor heard. Children are legally barred from such activities as gambling and drinking alcohol and from certain forms of entertainment, and they are consequently excluded from the venues where these activities take place. Elsewhere they are barred by convention, as in many restaurants, at adult parties or during certain adult conversations. Conversely, a whole range of special provisions are made for children: educational institutions that prepare them for adult life by removing them from it; clubs and organizations that cater for leisure pursuits quite separate from those of adults but that are all the same under adult control. Whole industries are geared to children, producing special clothes, toys and games and even wallpaper to adorn their bedrooms.

The details of such provisions are often criticized — complaints are made about advertisers' exploitation of children's desire for toys, heated debates rage around the extent to which the educational system meets their needs — but it is taken for granted that children's lives should be organized in a radically different manner from that of their elders. Underlying the laws and conventions which define the child's place in society are deep-rooted convictions about the nature of childhood, beliefs that brand a child as a particular sort of human being quite different from an adult.

Most of the special arrangements we make for children serve to emphasize this distinction. Their confinement in schools underlines their unfitness for the sort of work which is central to adult life. Children's clothes exaggerate their physical differentness; their toys and books and the songs and poems produced especially for them indicate that they are unable to enjoy adult leisure and cultural pursuits; nursery decor suggests that they are not expected to share the aesthetic tastes of the rest of society. So sharply are the distinctions between adult and child drawn that the two seem almost to belong to different species: adults are independent, children dependent; adults productive, children non-productive; adults work, children play; adults are involved in the serious business of life, childhood is supposed to be 'fun'. It is not simply that children are treated as people who have yet to learn the skills and conventions of adult life, but that they are regarded as beings of a different order with needs quite apart from those of the rest of the community.

Childhood is seen as a particular psychological state, so that 'child psychology' is considered quite distinct from adult psychology. (In fact the latter label is never used, for it is only the child's mental processes that are singled our for special expert attention.) Backed by the scientific rationale of psychology, the assumption that children are different is now accepted as a universal human truth and is shared by people with quite dissimilar views on childhood and child-rearing. While conservatives may argue that children need order and discipline and should learn to respect their elders, progressives advocate 'free expression'. While one side subjects children to indignities that would be insufferable to their elders, the other tolerates behaviour that would be completely unacceptable from adults. Both, however, expect children to behave differently, in accordance with a separate code of conduct from that accepted among adults.

Whatever pattern of child-rearing is adopted is usually justified by reference to children's special needs. Children's mental functioning is often discussed as if it were as far from adult comprehension as the mind of a cat or dog. The analogy could be extended, for in many ways children are treated much like household pets. I have noticed, for instance, that 'progressive' parents often have dogs as unruly as their children, and conservative disciplinarians expect both dogs and children to obey orders. It is often said that people keep pets as substitutes for children, but it may be that children are surrogate pets. Children are under the ownership and control of particular adults and to an extent they must accept whatever life their 'owners' or parents arrange for them. True, there are organizations that protect the interests of children and intervene where there is abuse or neglect — but equally there are societies for the protection of animals. Children are dressed to please adults, their activities are regulated by adults, they are expected to please others, to play cute, to show off their accomplishments as if they were a dog's new tricks. Adults discuss them in their presence as if they were not there, laugh at them when they are doing something they take quite seriously, talk down to them and pat them on the head or chuck them under the chin just as if they are stroking an animal. All this is seen as perfectly acceptable, even as being kind to children. If a child shows resentment at treatment that most adults would find thoroughly humiliating then she or he is cheeky, sulky or insolent.

All this suggests that childhood is not just a psychological state, but also a social status — and a very lowly one at that. Take one example: the frequency with which children are touched by adults. The amount of unsolicited physical contact people receive is a good indication of relative social position. It has been observed that bosses touch workers, men touch women and adults touch children much more than the other way around. To touch one's social superior without good reason is an act of insubordination. Think how frequently children are shaken off when they use touch to attract an adult's attention, and how that same adult can freely take hold of the child, adjust his or her hair, cut short his or her activities. Children have to put up with unwanted caresses when they would rather be doing something else, and are often victims of less gentle attention: research in the United States has shown that the majority of American parents not only hit their children regularly but believe they have the right to do so.

Children are a subordinate social group. They are economically unproductive and dependent in a society which values productivity and independence; they are denied full citizenship and adult legal rights and responsibilities. This is justified by the claim that their weakness and vulnerability, their need of protection and their lack of maturity all make them incapable of exercising rights, holding responsibility or making their own decisions. The adult always knows best.

Of course, someone who is relatively small and weak and who has not yet acquired the skills to survive socially and economically needs protection, support and guidance from the more experienced. But children are not encouraged to gain experience, to grow up, to mature into adult responsibilities and acquire rights and independence. They are kept dependent for much longer than necessary; a great deal of effort is spent in keeping children childish. Not being encouraged towards independence, they remain dependent; unused to looking after themselves, they stay vulnerable; having their smallest needs fulfilled by adults, they are often unable to perform simple tasks well within their capabilities. Children are frequently sent to school unable to dress themselves at an age when, in other societies and in earlier days of our own, they would be beginning to make a real contribution to the life and work of their community. If a child expresses interest in adult affairs or engages in adult pursuits it is thought unusual, even extraordinary. Children who behave like adults are regarded as at best amusing and at worst thoroughly obnoxious. If we were not so interested in nurturing immaturity, would the word 'precocious' have become an insult?

The sharp distinction we make between childhood and adulthood creates a gulf between the two that is bridged by that peculiar intermediate stage we call adolescence. Adolescents inhabit a strange in-between world, no longer children but still not adults, told to 'grow up' but denied the opportunity of participating in adult life. So childhood is prolonged, and young people are expected to become mature and prepare for adult society while remaining outside it. Most problems experienced by adolescents, not least the sexual ones, derive from the uncertainties and ambiguities of their situation, the result of the artificial dividing lines we have drawn between childhood and adulthood, as I shall show in chapter 7.

The anxiety and controversy surrounding the issue of children and sex must be seen in the context of this prolongation of childhood and the special status it is given. The concern to keep sex hidden from children stems from and is sometimes equated with the idea that childhood itself is in need of preservation, so that it is the sexual 'innocence' of children that above all else distinguishes them from adults. The pace at which children mature, especially sexually, is the object of much concern and speculation. Often one hears older people complaining that children grow up faster than they used to, or saying that children 'ought to be allowed to stay children' and enjoy their childhood, meaning that they should be shielded as far as possible from the realities of adult life, including sex. Although this suggests that people are aware that childhood may be changing, it also reveals a notion of the 'true nature' of the child — one thought to be threatened with violation and one that must be valued and cherished.

It would be difficult to define the 'true nature' of childhood, however, for there is little that can be said about it that is genuinely universal. Our children are asexual, apolitical, vulnerable, dependent, incapable of taking part in serious adult pursuits not because that is the way children naturally *are* but because that it the way they are treated. As I have hinted, the experience of childhood in other societies can be radically different.

I have already stressed the immense variation in human sexuality from culture to culture, and it is only to be expected that similar diversity will be found in other aspects of social life, including childhood. As with sexuality, we are dealing with basic biological facts which no society can ignore: in this case the pattern of growth from infancy to physical maturity. But these facts can be interpreted in a variety of different ways which in turn produce a variety of consequences for children's lives. All societies make some distinction between childhood and adulthood, but the means of drawing it and the degree of emphasis it bears vary widely. Some peoples make much of distinctions between the two, others little; in some societies children are expected to show extreme deference to their elders, in others none; sometimes the transition from 'child' to 'adult' is abrupt, sometimes gradual.

The activities and interests of children in other societies may contrast sharply with our ideas of what is natural or appropriate for them. We would find it strange for a boy of six or seven to be preoccupied with financial provision for his marriage, yet this is considered natural among the Tallensi. We would not expect a child of this age to be making a real contribution to the economic survival of the community, yet this is commonplace in many simpler societies. We would certainly not consider three-year-old children capable of fending for themselves, but this has been known in extreme conditions, for instance among the Ik, an African society about to disintegrate, where children beyond this age are no longer fed or cared for by adults. It is unusual for five-year-olds in our society to be fully aware of the facts of human sex and reproduction, but elsewhere this is normal.

Despite all the different forms of childhood that exist throughout the world, our society might be singled out as distinctly odd in some aspects of its treatment of children. In few simpler societies are children kept so much apart from the adult social world, rarely do they have so small a range of contacts with people outside their own age group, and seldom are they as dependent on particular adults as they are in most Western societies. There is no need for separate educational facilities when the young have ample opportunity to learn by participating in adult tasks. There is no need for toys to develop infants' minds and skills when they are constantly stimulated by the activities of those around them, or for toys and games for older children when they are allowed to enjoy adult festivities and leisure pursuits. Children do not need to be so tied to their parents when work and leisure are organized on a more communal basis and where they are encouraged to learn the skills necessary for independence. Evidence from other cultures shows us that what we consider 'natural' for children is by no means universal and fixed.

The anthropological evidence suggests that there are certain features of technologically simple, small scale societies that allow children to be more thoroughly integrated into adult social life than is possible in modern industrial societies. These simpler societies may appear as different from each other as they are from our own, but despite the great range of social organization and cultural life among them they share certain important features: work and leisure involve the same small groups of people, and there is little or no distinction between the private world of home and leisure and the public world of the workplace. This raises the possibility that somewhere in our own past, before the beginnings of capitalism and industrialization, when communities were smaller and work centred more on the household, childhood might have been a rather different institution from what it has become today.

But reconstructing the history of childhood is no easy task. In the first place, sources are few and scattered. As the historian Peter Laslett has pointed out, there was a far higher proportion of children in pre-industrial society, but these large numbers are invisible in historical records. Demographic data becomes more sparse and less accurate the further back in history one delves. A few diaries tell us something about childhood in earlier times, but only about the more prosperous sections of society. For example, Heroard's account of the childhood of Louis XIII of France tells us much about the life of a royal child in the early seventeenth century, but his lot must have been totally different from that of a peasant at that time. Of the childhood of ordinary folk we know little, except what we hear from such individuals as social reformers in Tudor England or zealous country clergymen in seventeenth-century France, and these accounts are needless to say somewhat distorted. Clues are also provided by representations of children in early art — their presence or absence in crowd scenes, as well as the portraits of them — but here care is needed. For example, does the fact that children were depicted as small adults mean that most people viewed them like that, or was it simply an artistic convention?

Despite the paucity of sources, they do when pieced together provide enough evidence to demonstrate that childhood has indeed changed. In interpreting them, however, we should avoid romanticizing the lives of our ancestors and imagining that there was a golden age of childhood at some point in the past. We should equally avoid the other extreme, that of seeing history as uninterrupted progress, its every change an improvement.

Care should also be taken not to overemphasize the differences between pre-modern and modern society and imagine contrasts that do not exist. Although considerable change has occurred, it is change within a particular society and cultural

31

heritage. People sometimes think, for example, that our forebears were all peasants living in three-generation families, tied to the land and surviving solely by subsistence farming. Although this may have been true in parts of eastern Europe, it was not typical of the rest of it and certainly not of England. Many features of Western society that are thought distinctly modern, and that have profound effects on childhood, seem to have their origins in medieval times or even earlier. For most of western Europe the family has long been based on the small unit of parents and children. Although the population was predominantly rural, by no means everyone was engaged in agriculture and, at least in most of Britain, wage labour and individual private property developed early.

These continuities between the past and present, however, go hand in hand with certain discontinuities. Production, whether agricultural or otherwise, did tend to be small scale and based on the household if not on the family. Children began work early in their lives, and a form of wage labour made it possible for them to cease to be dependent on their parents much earlier than they can today. Few special arrangements were made for children; once they were beyond infancy they were not thought to have many needs different from those of their elders, and it was not considered necessary to shield them from the realities of adult life, however harsh they might be,

The path to adulthood in medieval society involved passing through infancy, childhood and youth, but these three stages were not the same as they are today. Infants were neglected and maltreated by modern standards, childhood was a much briefer phase and youth began earlier and ended later than our adolescence. Children were generally not so tightly enmeshed in their families and were far more a part of the larger community than they are today.

Infancy was a precarious time; only half the babies born could be expected to survive until their first birthday. Since they might be only temporary visitors to the world of the living, they were not so central to family life as they have since become. In colonial times, frontier parents in North America would often leave a new baby unnamed for several months lest they waste a good name on someone who might not survive. Although early baptism had for long been the rule on the other side of the Atlantic (favourite names were recycled if their original owners had not needed them for long), infants were not seen as very important and they received little attention or affection. Whether children were neglected because adults detached themselves from beings who might soon be dead, or whether death was a straightforward consequence of neglect, is debatable. It is impossible to establish cause and effect: probably the two factors reinforced each other. What we would now judge as maltreatment was associated with indifference rather than calculated cruelty. Some of the practices associated with the high infant mortality rate, such as swaddling and its attendant lack of hygiene and the system of wetnursing, seem to have been more a matter of custom than individual attitudes.

Little is known of children's lives between their emerging from the wholly marginal state of infancy and the age of about seven. At this time most would have been living with their parents, but in a household which might include unrelated youths and adults, though it was unlikely to contain any other relatives except their brothers and sisters. Since no special provision was made for children of this age we must assume that they simply fitted into the life of the household and the community as best they could. By the age of seven they were considered legally responsible for their own actions, and in Tudor Britain children as young as this could be (and were) hanged for capital offences. They would also be expected to be making a substantial economic contribution. In 1724 the writer Daniel Defoe stated that children of four or five should be able to earn their daily bread.

Somewhere between the age of seven and fourteen the majority of children would leave home to enter another household as living-in servants, thus abandoning childhood and entering youth. As servants, they would not only be involved in domestic service, but often apprenticed in a trade or employed in agriculture. They did not live 'below stairs' but became part of the family household under the control of its head. Not only the rich employed servants; minor craftsmen and landholders would often have one or two young people living under their roofs as servants. Some historians have suggested that this system provided a means of correcting inbalances in the supply and demand of home-bred labour, so that those families without enough offspring to do their work would take in servants from those with children surplus to their needs. So at different times, depending on the number and age of its children, a family might both hire servants and provide them for others. This seems to have been true of some sections of the population at least, but evidence also suggests that a more direct exchange of children also went on, some families parting with their own offspring and simultaneously taking in others. The early age at which children left home may have been not simply the result of economic necessity, but also what was thought the right and proper way to set young people on the road to adulthood. Among the gentry and aristocracy it seems to have been thought an essential part of a young person's education, teaching them more of the morals and values of their society. Perhaps a similar attitude motivated those lower down the social scale. In any case, this early departure from the parental home seems to have been the lot of most young people in Britain and many elsewhere in Europe, though not everywhere. One Italian observer of English society in the early sixteenth century clearly found the practice neither normal nor acceptable and thought it symptomatic of the 'want of affection' in the English, feeling that it amounted to very harsh treatment.

From our present position it would be easy to agree, but we should remember that a sixteenth-century child may not have found separation as disturbing as many twentieth-century English and American children would. Children in pre-modern times were much less cosseted and protected and would have been tougher and more independent; having had contact with a wider range of people outside their family they would also have been less emotionally dependent on their parents. (Indeed, the snippets of advice on child-rearing that have come down to us from that time suggest that emotional dependence was strongly discouraged.)

The period which began with this move from home lasted until young people reached their late twenties. During this time they received board and lodging from their masters or patrons and often money wages too. Among the upper classes this arrangement offered young people opportunities to further their career or marriage prospects by broadening their range of social contacts. Usually people were bound to this service for a set period of years. Most could not escape until they had come into an inheritance, acquired the skills and resources to set up in a craft or trade, or, at the bottom of the hierarchy, acquired a cottage or become a day labourer. Marriage generally occurred at this stage; earlier it would have been impractical (because of lack of money) or impossible (because of the legal bond of apprenticeship). Marriage, the mark of full adult status that followed upon economic and social independence, took place rather later in life than is usual today.

Youth was a period of semi-independence. Parental control was exchanged for that of master or patron, but many young servants and apprentices seem to have enjoyed some freedom outside the household, their leisure activities governed by groups of their fellows. In villages these youth groups played a leading part in organizing communal gatherings and seasonal festivities. By and large youth seems to have been more closely defined and bounded than is our modern equivalent, adolescence.

Children and young people were once much more closely integrated into the working and social life of the community as a whole. Their education did not take place in separate institutions and they prepared for adult life by participating in it. Apprenticeship was the nearest thing to schooling that most of them experienced; what formal education existed was mostly in the hands of the clergy. Apart from those entering religious orders, few but the wealthy had an education in our sense. Teaching, where it was given, was not tailored to the needs of children. No textbooks were produced for them; they learnt from whatever books or manuscripts were available to adults. Nor was there any notion of grading — teaching particular skills at a particular age or in a particular order. It was not unusual for people of widely varying ages to be taught the same things together, and early schools were not organized in grades or classes. In the sixteenth century the famous English public school, Eton, had only one large schoolroom which served all purposes. Under these circumstances it was no great disadvantage to begin one's education late; at the same time, precocity was not unusual. Children of the more privileged members of society often made very rapid progress in their studies. John Evelyn, an English gentleman, claimed that his son Richard could read English, French and Latin at the age of two and a half and that, at the age of five, he had 'a strange passion for Greeke'.

So work and education provided little basis for differentiating between children and adults, and the same was true of leisure and entertainment. Here children and youths shared the activities of their elders. While they may have had their own roles to play, they were not excluded, nor sent off early to bed while adults continued to make merry. The folk tales and songs which have come down to us as fairy stories and nursery rhymes were not originally reserved for children but were part of an oral tradition shared by all, and children's party games, such as blind man's buff, were once played by adults, even among the aristocracy. Poorer children took part in the seasonal round of village festivals and celebrations; aristocratic youngsters participated in gambling, sport, masques, dances and music. Just as these children could be far advanced in learning, so they were in the more general social arts and graces. By the time Louis XIII was two years old he was playing tennis and mall, being taught to play the violin and beginning to learn adult dances.

In many ways medieval children do seem to have been treated as miniature adults. They were dressed in adult clothes — according to their sex and class rather than their age — and shared in the lives of their elders. They were not thought to need special provisions in work, play or education. Although lacking the legal status of adults they were held legally responsible for their actions and were subject to the same penalties as adults if they broke the law. So, while childhood definitely had a subordinate social status, it was not regarded as a psychological state. It is this change in emphasis from status to state which has marked the rise of the modern institution of childhood.

It is difficult to pinpoint the exact origin of the change, but it began to be evident among the more prosperous sections of society by the end of the sixteenth century, corresponding with the rise to ascendancy of the capitalist classes and the accompanying changes in family life. In England, where the individualistic values characteristic of capitalism had been prevalent for some time, families were already closing in around their children. The upper classes had relegated their servants to their own quarters and began to show an increasing desire for privacy in their family life. Male children started to receive formal education instead of being sent into the households of patrons, though their sisters continued to follow this course into the seventeenth century, and among the common people this service or apprenticeship persisted for much longer. So in

38

effect upper-class boys seems to have been the first children to be singled out as such. It was some time before their sisters were affected by these changes, and even longer before the lives of the majority of lower-class children were substantially altered. This pattern of change was no chance product of historical accident: the first 'specialized children' were being trained as the first specialized entrepreneurs in a society more and more centred on trade and manufacture.

Some of the early instances of change in the nature of childhood may seem relatively insignificant, but they do show that children were beginning to be singled out for special treatment. For the first time children's dress was differentiated from adults'. Initially this affected only boys under the age of about seven, but gradually it spread to older children and girls. Special clothes for children long remained the preserve of the middle and upper classes. It is interesting that the earliest children's costumes were copied from adult fashions of previous generations, and later they borrowed elements from working-class clothes. Just as children were bequeathed clothes that adults judged too out-of-date or 'common' for themselves, so games, rhymes and stories once enjoyed by all came to be seen as too unsophisticated, suitable only for children or the common people. The first English nursery-rhyme book was published in 1744, and by this time old folk tales were also being written down and printed in a form thought suitable for children.

In the meantime there had been a growing concern with the special needs of children; the first books on paediatrics began to appear in the sixteenth century. Age-grading in schools gradually became accepted and children began to be taught from textbooks specially prepared for them. The children of the established upper classes and the rising bourgeoisie found their education extended — where once the age of entrance to the English universities had been twelve, by the seventeenth century it had risen to fifteen. As the family began to close in around them, with the exclusion of servants and the creation of greater privacy, children became more important to it, indeed its very focus. Wetnursing and swaddling began to disappear and infants received more attention and affection. Older children were kept within the home, sent away, if at all, only for formal education. Boarding schools were less popular on the continent than in Britain, but even when boys did go away to school the break from home was milder than under the old patronage and apprenticeship system.

The lives of children lower down the social scale changed more slowly. They continued to share in the working and social lives of adults of their class. Not for them the distinctive clothing or formal education: the former required affluence and the latter was long considered unsuitable for children of humble origins. They continued to be prepared for adult life through work. As the servant system declined and employment opportunities became centred on urban areas it was largely young people who pioneered the move to the towns. In the new industrial era children continued to work, but in the factory rather than the household, and their wages long remained crucial to the upkeep, even the survival, of their families.

It was a long time before children were barred from such work. In the United States at the turn of the century well over two million children under fifteen were full-time labourers. In New York four-year-olds worked sixteen hours a day sorting beads or rolling cigars while in Southern cotton mills five-year-old girls worked the night shift. In Britain it was not until the middle of the nineteenth century that protective legislation began to exclude children from productive work, and there was no compulsory education for all until 1870. The appalling conditions under which children worked did not alone force these changes, though they did, combined with Victorian middle-class sentimentality about the child, motivate individual reformers. Economic circumstances were changing and the demand for child labour decreased; at the same time fear of the 'dangerous poor' became more pronounced among the prosperous classes, and they felt a pressing need to control working-class children and youths, to impose middle-class standards upon them. To a large extent the modern institution of childhood was forced on working-class people rather than freely adopted by them, although many soon came to view a comfortable family life and the 'protection' of children within it as a symbol of higher living standards and a goal to aim for.

Social change is usually accompanied by ideological change — the development of new values and attitudes to justify new patterns of life. So changes in the pattern of children's lives was accompanied by the rise of particular images of the child, notions of the nature of childhood and ideals of childish behaviour. As childhood began to be defined as a special category, two images arose that have never quite vanished from the popular imagination, aptly dubbed by sociologist Arlene Skolnick the 'demoniac' and 'innocent' child.

When attention was first focused on the special

nature of the child it was in the context of the social upheaval of the Reformation and the Counter-Reformation. Puritans, on the one side, and Jesuits, on the other, became concerned with educational reform and the spiritual well-being of children as part of a wider campaign against moral laxity. To them the child was corrupt, tainted by original sin, an un-civilized being whose demoniac nature had to be tamed. The aim of education was to break the spirit of these creatures, and their advice to parents and educators recommended punitive measures to counter children's naturally evil natures.

This view became modified in the Romantic era of the late eighteenth and early nineteenth centuries. The child as savage became identified with the 'Noble Savage' (also an invention of the time), and civiliza-tion was seen as the embodiment of corruption rather than a bastion against it. Children were innocent of the sin of the world and required protection from it. This Romantic image fostered a gentler approach to child-rearing and a sentimental attitude towards children. But in reality this change in attitude had less effect on children's lives than we might expect, since the two images could be used to justify similar treat-ment, in particular children's exclusion from adult society.

In the course of time, with the rise of scientific rationalism in the nineteenth century, the new discipline of psychology was formed, and new theories of child development emerged that were partly super-imposed upon, and partly replaced, the earlier religious and Romantic imagery. The new theories claimed as their basis a new criterion of universal truth: the god Science. Developmental theories of one kind or another have been with us ever since; their proponents include such well-known figures as Freud and Piaget. Childhood was redefined as a set of 'natural' paths of development: children passed through various pre-determined stages en route to adulthood. Despite all the historical and anthropological evidence to the contrary, these theorists claim that they have at last uncovered the true nature of childhood, and their theories have made their way into almost all our lives via the (often contradictory) advice of 'experts' and child-rearing manuals, and the practices of teachers and welfare professionals.

The historical transition from childhood as social status to childhood as psychological state is now complete. But children are still treated as social inferiors, and it may not be that child-rearing has become less authoritarian, as many people think, but that we are more subtle in the exercise of authority, that our techniques have changed from open force to subtle manipulation.

All these changes in child-rearing practices and images of childhood have affected our attitudes to children and sex and our perceptions of children's sexuality. Before children were singled out as creatures with special needs there was little reason to conceal sex from them, and before the development of modern, private domestic arrangements there was little opportunity to do so.

In medieval times, concealment would simply not have been practicable. Most people did not enjoy the luxury of privacy, and even the living arrangements of the aristocracy did not prevent children stumbling across copulating couples. It is probable that up to the early seventeenth century children of all social classes were aware of the physical facts of sex when they were little more than toddlers. Some historians have suggested that this produced sexually maladjusted adults, and much has been made of Louis XIII's early exposure to sex as a cause of his adult sexual and emotional problems. Little Louis slept in the same room as his married servants — who appear to have been quite uninhibited in his presence — and he was encouraged to take an interest in sex and to play sexual games with his sister. None of his contemporaries, however, seemed to think this unusual, so unless one wants to claim that the entire aristocratic population of seventeenth-century France was sexually unbalanced, it is unwise to infer too much from it. In any case, more recent child-rearing practices can hardly be said to produce adults free of sexual problems.

Whatever the consequences of this state of affairs, it was not to continue for much longer — at least, not among the upper classes. Most historians agree that the seventeenth century was the turning point. Moralists began to campaign against common habits such as multiple occupancy of beds and bedrooms, the lax attitudes towards children's sex games, and the practice of leaving children in the company of servants, who came to be seen as a corrupting influence. As these new ideas became accepted, changes occurred in the tuition of, and in the amusements deemed suitable for, children.

At a time when children were not shielded from the reality of sex, there was no reason to exclude them from any other form of contact with it. Games and entertainments were seldom restricted to one age group, and sexual references were common in the songs, jokes and stories that children heard. Those children who received formal education would encounter sexual themes as a matter of course:

bawdy rhymes and riddles were used as teaching aids, and the accepted classics included much erotic material and a great deal of sexual humour. During the late sixteenth and early seventeenth centuries, however, many traditional texts were withdrawn from the curriculum, some to reappear in expurgated form. The Jesuits, for example, decreed that Terence was not fit for children to read and subsequently produced their own version, described as 'Comedies of Terence made very decent while changing very little'. A similarly censored version was produced in Britain.

The history of the fairy tale provides a further illustration of this trend. Fairy tales were not at first intended specifically for children, but by the time they came to be written down they had lost their appeal to more sophisticated adults since they were no longer so relevant to their lives. They came to be regarded as quaint curiosities fit only for peasants, servants and children. The old versions contained a good deal of explicit sex, preserved in some of the printed collections. Modern parents might be rather alarmed if they found their children reading an authentic edition of Grimms' fairy tales. As the stories were originally recorded, the Sleeping Beauty was awakened not by a kiss but by rape, and the Frog Prince, admitted into the Princess's room in amphibian form, regained his naked human shape in time to spend the night in her bed; later 'The wedding arrangements were hastened that the christening might not follow too soon.' Material like this was quickly removed from the versions that were prepared for children. Since then we have passed through a stage of our history when sex was considered unseemly even as a topic in adult literature. Modern times are more liberal, but still not where children are concerned.

These changes reflected the images of children which were developing over this period, culminating in a notion of childish 'innocence' that has come to be equated with sexual ignorance. There is some evidence that the idea that children are sexually innocent already existed in early modern times, but in a form very different from that current today. Some historians have suggested that the reason why children of Louis XIII's generation were so casually exposed to sex was because they were not thought to have any sexual needs or feelings. It was acceptable to talk and joke with children about sex and play sexual games with them because they were oblivious to any erotic significance, and greater propriety was unnecessary until they became adult. So their innocence, far from needing protection, was thought itself to protect them from immorality.

In the era of the demoniac child the idea of original sin was closely associated with sex; the child's sexuality was an integral part of the beast that had to be kept at bay. Exposure to sexuality was dangerous because it aroused a part of human nature best kept down and might prevent children from overcoming their inborn sinful urges. When the idea of the innocent child arose it provided a new rationale for keeping sex from children: to preserve their innocence rather than to counter their guilt.

Thus it was that opposing attitudes justified similar trends in child-rearing. Children were taught to observe standards of modesty and decency from an early age and were no longer allowed free access to sexual knowledge. The eighteenth century saw the beginnings of the campaign against infantile masturbation. The Church had always regarded this activity as sinful in adults but had been tolerant of it in children. Medical opinion had previously regarded it as beneficial in moderation though harmful in excess. But now clergy and physicians united in condemning masturbation, viewing it as the cause of all manner of moral and physical ills. From then on children had to be guarded from their own desires as well as others'. The idea that any contact with sex sullies childhood innocence has been with us ever since, as has the spectre of the demonaic child and the fear that children may not be as innocent as we would like. Hence the Victorians combined a cloying sentimentality towards children with severe physical punishment of childish misdeeds and vicious suppression of any apparently sexual behaviour.

We should not imagine that these changes took place overnight or that they affected all sections of society at once. It was some time before the majority achieved living standards that made such 'protection' possible. As late as the nineteenth century this problem vexed the 'respectable' sectors of society, who feared for the morals of the poor. The British philanthropists and reformers who concentrated their efforts on the plight of children were often more worried about the moral consequences of their living and working conditions than about their physical suffering. Overcrowded housing particularly alarmed them. The Reverend Andrew Mearns, in his famous tract *The Bitter Cry of Outcast London*, said that under such circumstances, 'no form of vice or sexuality causes surprise'. Lord Shaftesbury, voicing similar anxieties in the House of Lords, spoke coyly of 'every social and domestic necessity' having to be performed in one crowded room. The fight to ban child labour in the mines gained much support by virtue of middle-class horror at the thought of people of all ages and both sexes working together semi-naked. The report of the Royal Commission on the subject, published in 1842, made it clear that while the physical consequences of such work for children were deplorable, the moral consequences were even worse. It is full of references to 'the immoral effects' of such employment and to the 'savage rudeness' of children's upbringing, and hints at the dreadful effects: they 'grew accustomed to obscene language, vice, debauchery, and knew no impropriety in them'. Clearly the Victorian conscience was highly sensitive to the idea that the innocence of a whole class of children was being corrupted.

Most people are still ready to express horror and outrage at any threat to children's innocence, but now concern has shifted from anxieties about their moral and spiritual well-being to the psychological effects of early contact with sex. There are new ways of rationalizing the need to keep them in ignorance, but the old ideas have never been completely eradicated — simply incorporated into a more 'scientific' way of thinking. The belief that children are asexual is now rarer and sex itself is less often regarded as sinful, yet the taboo on children and sex is still firmly entrenched and sexuality still carries the tag 'for adults only'. It is these attitudes, the ways in which we seek to conceal sex from children and the effects of this concealment that I will now go on to explore.

4

For Adults Only

The taboo that serves to keep sex hidden from children is one of the most powerful in modern society. It is enforced in both public and private life, through formal legislation and through informal — but nonetheless potent — rules governing what may be said or done in a child's presence. The power of this taboo is most evident when it is broken, when a teacher is discovered revealing the 'facts of life' to five-year-olds or when an early evening television programme depicts sexual acts. Children are thought to be vulnerable and sexuality a threat to their well-being.

The rationale for the taboo is the need to protect children from aspects of life that are thought to be harmful to them. But any taboo is more than just a set of rules; it also involves complex emotional reactions. The desire to conceal sex from children reflects not only our ideas of what is good and bad for them, but also adult fears and anxieties about sexuality. Why, for example, do less than half of British and American parents discuss sexual matters, even with their adolescent children? Is it because they wish to avoid harming them, or because they find it difficult to talk about sex, or because they are unable to accept their children's emerging sexuality? In the Victorian era, sex was thought so grave a danger that infants had their hands tied to their sides or clamped to the edge of their cots to prevent them abusing themselves. In the early decade of this century, especially in the United States, clitoridectomy was a popular 'cure' for small girls who masturbated. Was this violence genuinely provoked by what seemed like a threat to children, or were adults simply projecting their own inhibitions? We may have become more humane in our treatment of children and more subtle in controlling their sexual development, but it is still considered our duty to protect them from sex and our right to impose our own morality on them in the process.

A good place to detect the taboo in action is in the kind of entertainment selected as suitable for children. Sex is prominent among the themes thought too disturbing for children, but others are also treated with caution, notably violence. It is interesting to compare attitudes to the two to see some of the inconsistences in the way adults think about children and sex.

Whether at the cinema or on television screens at home, children are likely to witness far more violence than sex in the entertainment provided for them. Violent death on a large scale is not seen as a threat to their supposedly delicate psyches, but the most gentle act of sex apparently is. Only a few parents worry about their children watching old westerns or war movies in which Indians or outlaws, Germans or Japanese predictably bite the dust in their hundreds. As long as it is good clean death without too much explicit detail of blood and gore, all is well. Good clean sex is, however, out of the question, and most adults would be more at ease if their children were watching death scenes than acts of love. It seems absurd that genocide is a fit subject for family entertainment while even the sight of animals mating has been known to prevent a film being granted a U certificate (i.e., suitable for children) in Britain.

These absurdities are more comprehensible if we take a sceptical view of avowed aims of censorship. The theory and practice of this form of censorship show some interesting inconsistencies which suggest that underlying the claim of protecting the young from material that might frighten, upset or confuse them are quite different intentions: to protect not the child's mental health, but a certain type of morality. Take violence, for example: to glorify it is more widely accepted than to portray its grim results. Campaigners against sex and violence on the large and small screens often base their case against violence on its presumed effects on younger viewers. They fear it might promote a callous acceptance of real violence and inspire acts of teenage aggression. One of Britain's foremost agitators takes this view and yet has also said that too much explicit detail in war films might put young people off violence, with the deplorable effect of sapping the nation's will to fight. This concern is less with the psychological well-being of immature audiences than with harnessing their aggression to particular ends. Not surprisingly, there are similar contradictions when people try to justify the censoring of sexual scenes. People fear that explicit portrayals of eroticism might mar healthy sexual development, and at the same time they worry that it might lead to too healthy an interest in sex and thus threaten the established morality.

Not all sexual material is filtered out of children's entertainment. Though sexuality is clearly marked out as an adult preserve, as we have seen, and erotic films and books are labelled 'adult entertainment', its opposite, 'family entertainment', is not always empty of any sexual import. While its hallmark is the absence of any explicit reference to sex, it may use innuendo. This is the basis of much humour in comedy films and television shows and is typical of that prime example of family entertainment, the Christmas pantomime. Jokes based on veiled references to sex or on *double entendre* are of course aimed at the adult section of the audience and assumed to pass over the children's heads. But children know when something is being hidden from them or when they don't get the joke, and they will often laugh so as not to seem stupid. They are learning that this thing that they cannot understand is somehow rather naughty and dirty, and that this is why it is funny. They are thus learning negative attitudes to sex even before they know what it is. That children are exposed to this sort of message, but denied access to anything that would allow them to make sense of it, illustrates once more that it is adults' morality not children's sensitivity that is being protected.

Even more evidence can be found in the censorship on behalf of adolescents — acknowledged as sexually aware but not yet adult enough to select their own entertainment. In Britain young people over the age of fourteen are admitted to films with the certificate AA, but they must be eighteen before they are allowed to view films in the adult X category. Sexuality may be depicted in both types of film, but with some interesting differences. Sexual intercourse may be shown in X films, but is only implied in AA films.

Sexual intercourse in any other position than with the man on top has only recently become acceptable for adult audiences, and is still not even implied in movies seen by fourteen- to eighteen-year-olds; homosexual lovemaking may not be shown to this younger group though its existence may be admitted. If there is any explanation it must run as follows: young people are allowed to know that sex happens, but not to see it; they may be shown shots which tell them a lot about how it is done provided that they are given no hint that the man does not have to be on top; they can discover that homosexuals and lesbians exist, but must not be aware of how they make love. These sorts of distinctions have nothing at all to do with protecting young people's interests but a good deal to do with maintaining traditional sexual attitudes and practices.

If the real purpose of this selective censorship is to avoid upsetting children, then many films made specifically for them would be banned and Disney Productions would have gone bankrupt years ago. Anyone who can recall their earliest visits to the cinema can usually remember some harrowing experiences. I have vivid recollections of sobbing throughout most of *The Lady and the Tramp*, greatly distressed by the unjust treatment of the Tramp, and of being so terrified by the forest fire in *Bambi* that I cowered under the seat. Some years later my younger sister, then about four years old, was taken to see *Mary Poppins*. She had to be removed from the cinema screaming 'Don't like it!' at the top of her voice, and was still in tears when my father brought her home. I cannot imagine either of us being so disturbed by watching sex on the screen, though we might have been curious or perhaps bored. At the age of fifteen, freed from British censorship by living in the Far East, I saw many films that were given X certificates or banned altogether back home and that would, no doubt, have been considered most unsuitable for a girl of my tender years. None of these films caused me any anxiety and they certainly did me far less mental damage than *Bambi* had done ten years before.

Film censorship would make no sense at all were it not just one of many means by which we deliberately conceal sex from children. They do not find any mention of sex in the books they read, the films they see or the television programmes they watch; they are kept out of conversation about sex, prevented from observing sexual acts, rarely see adults unclad and even have dolls that are made without genitals or nipples. If they somehow manage to frame questions about sex, they are usually met with an evasive, if not downright hostile, response. On average, children have little understanding of sex and almost no opportunity to find out about it. Not until they approach adolescence are they initiated into this secret knowledge; only then can they begin to make sense of those fragments that have slipped through the net woven by adult inhibitions.

Until they reach the age when they are considered old enough to receive sexual knowledge, children are thought to be incapable of coping with it, as though it demanded a special kind of maturity. It is here that the idea that children are a 'special' category of people meets the notion that sexuality is a 'special' area of life. If children were not so sharply differentiated from adults, so segregated from adult life, we would not be able to judge certain knowledge or behaviour inappropriate for them, nor so easily hide things from them. The reasons why this particular form of everyday experience is concealed from children lie in our attitudes to sexuality itself — the conventions of secrecy and privacy that surround it, the habit of cutting it off from the rest of our daily lives and keeping our sexual relationships exclusively to ourselves. Children therefore have an incomplete picture of the adult world: one important facet of it is always turned away from them. As a result they cannot learn about sexuality gradually, in the same way that they learn about the rest of the world they live in.

But this is not true everywhere. In societies where children are more fully part of the social life of their elders, and where there is a more open attitude to sex, it is rarely possible to pinpoint a time when they first become aware of it: here sex is not a secret kept by the adult community. An anecdote told by the anthropologist Malinowski about the Trobriand Islanders illustrates this very different attitude. He was discussing an 'obscene' subject with a group of men when the small daughter of one of them joined the group. Malinowski, taking the usual Western attitude, suggested that they should send the girl away so that they could finish their conversation. The Islanders saw no reason to do that. The child, they said, was not prone to gossip and would not repeat anything confidential that she overheard. They were concerned not that the conversation was unsuitable for the ears of a child, but rather whether the girl could be trusted to keep any secrets they might exchange in the course of it.

As I have shown in chapter 3, the desire to hide sex from children has not always been present in our own society. Our current secrecy is usually explained in terms of children's inability to understand sexual matters. It is generally believed that, firstly, sexuality is beyond young children's comprehension — they lack what psychologists call the 'cognitive capacity' to cope with it. Secondly, the argument goes, as they cannot understand it they would find it frightening and disturbing. But these assumptions do not stand up to close scrutiny. Children have no difficulty in understanding other kinds of sensual pleasure, so why should this particular sort be beyond them? Why should an activity that is physically enjoyable and has the added bonus of expressing attraction and affection be seen as disturbing? There is no factual basis for either of these assumptions. In other cultures (such as those of the Mbuti, !Kung or Trobrianders) who have a more positive and less secretive attitude to sexuality, children have no difficulty in assimilating the sexual information at their disposal. They learn early that sex is pleasurable, incorporate it unselfconsciously into their games, and, as they mature, gradually replace play by more adult forms of sexual expression.

Most children in our culture, however, are reared in a more conventional manner and encounter our more usual attitudes to sex, full of paradoxes and contradictions. Most adults would agree that sex is potentially pleasurable and enjoyable, yet they see it as posing a threat to children. They would probably prefer children to grow up thinking of sex as natural rather than squalid and dirty, yet they take great pains to hide it from them. Even when the secret is revealed, it is shrouded in so much customary modesty and morality that it is hardly likely to seem natural.

Even parents who take a more liberal line often treat knowledge about sex as different in kind from any other. A common claim is that children will ask

56

questions when they are ready to know. Their questions should be answered honestly, not evaded, for this could be damaging — but to tell them before they ask is also seen as dangerous, as 'forcing' it on them. This ignores the fact that children are constantly receiving unsolicited (and often unwanted) information from adults: the entire education system operates in this way. Again the implication is that sexuality is a subject unique in needing a great deal of caution and sensitivity if it is not to disturb the child.

The idea that children should only be told about sex when they ask is one of the main reasons why many parents never say anything at all about it. One of the most common excuses is 'They didn't seem interested' or 'They never asked about it'. Parental honesty can also only work if children ask the right questions — something that demands some prior knowledge of the subject. If a child has never seen an elephant s/he is unlikely to ask why it has a trunk — and children who have no idea about sex are just as unlikely to express curiosity about it.

I can draw a parallel here between our belief that children need protection against the ill effects of sexuality, and 'pollution beliefs' in simpler societies, beliefs that define contact between sex and other activities as contaminating and dangerous. Just as other peoples are careful to avoid any association between sex and eating, or are aware of the dangers of the sexual powers of one sex over the other, so we are anxious to avoid any meeting between sex and children — for us, the ultimate defilement.

Pollution beliefs, though, are rarely as irrational as they seem. As the anthropologist Mary Douglas has pointed our, they often serve to reinforce social arrangements that are somehow precarious. Our taboos surrounding children and sex are one of the means by which we maintain the distinctions between childhood and adulthood, and are also part of a morality which defines marriage as the only legitimate basis for sex. Both the critics and the defenders of the family see it as the backbone of society and any threat to it a sign of the breakdown of society. Freer forms of sexual relationships and different patterns of child-rearing might pose such a threat. Certainly those people who defend our sexual taboos most vociferously are apt to express the fear that breaking them will sweep away the family and all social order with it.

There may, however, be a more immediate and valid reason for our concern to protect children from sex, for in a real sense it *is* dangerous to them. In our society sexuality has a darker side that is closely connected with violence, aggression and exploitation. The words that name sexual acts and organs are also used as terms of abuse. We are brought up to think of sex in terms not so much of mutual pleasure but of activity and passivity, dominance and submission, something one person does to another. Usually it is men who are the 'doers' and women the 'done to', for men are brought up to view sexual conquest as a way of proving themselves, asserting their masculinity and demonstrating their dominance. Women are the usual victims, but once sex is seen as using someone else and associated with power and dominance, children too become targets. So sex can be a threat to children, one against which they do need shielding.

This may help to explain adult fears about children and sex, but it hardly makes our behaviour look any more rational. Keeping children in ignorance of sexuality does not protect them; it is more likely to make them more vulnerable. Telling them not to talk to strangers or accept lifts or sweets is not enough to keep them from danger. When children are molested it is usually not by strangers but by neighbours, family friends and relatives, people who have the chance to gain the child's confidence and to be alone with him or her. Even when the molester is a stranger, he can often easily persuade a young child that he is not; children are taught to defer to adults and accept what they say, which renders them powerless in situations that might harm them. The warnings children are usually given serve little purpose other than to fill them with vague fears of monstrous people out to do terrible things.

Whatever other fragments of knowledge children might have about sex, it is unlikely that they will connect them with these cautions: they simply do not know what they are being warned against. Nor have they any means of reading the signs that indicate the possibility of a sexual approach, or of anticipating what might happen. Since they cannot see the threat, they have little opportunity of making an escape before it is carried out.

An excellent fictional account of the dangers of such ignorance, particularly for girls who might appear more mature than they actually are, is provided in Carson McCullers's novel *The Member of the Wedding*. Her heroine, twelve-year-old Frankie (or F. Jasmine, as she is calling herself at the time), encounters a soldier whom she agrees to meet for a 'date'. She is trying to appear like a 'grown girl', and realizes that the soldier's invitation means he has accepted her new image. She knows that dating carries prestige for older girls, but has only observed it from the outside. Her sexual ignorance means that she knows neither the rules of the game nor the stakes of play. When the soldier invites her up to his room, she does not understand what it might mean nor has she learnt the usual tactics for beating a retreat. Unwilling or unable to abandon the role in which she has cast herself, she has unwittingly given the impression that she is sexually available.

F. Jasmine did not want to go upstairs, but she did not know how to refuse. It was like going into a fair booth, or a fair ride, that once having entered you cannot leave until the exhibition or ride is finished. Now it was the same with this soldier, this date. She could not leave until it ended. The soldier was waiting at the foot of the stairs and, unable to refuse, she followed after him.

She is now wary. Events have turned in a direction her idea of dating has not led her to expect, and the soldier no longer lives up to the romantic, heroic image she has of his profession. But not only is she taking a roller-coaster ride from which it is impossible to escape, she is doing so blindfolded with no idea of what will happen next. As her uneasiness grows, she makes to leave the room.

But as she passed the soldier, he grasped her skirt and, limpened by fright, she was pulled down beside him on the bed. She felt his arms around her and smelled his sweaty shirt. He was not rough, but it was crazier than if he had been rough — in a second she was paralyzed by horror.

Frankie is resourceful enough to bite the soldier, hit him over the head with a water pitcher and make a quick exit down the fire escape. A girl like this, knowing about glamour and romance but not about the sex that accompanies them, is vulnerable precisely because of her ignorance. Even after the event Frankie can only make sense of it as 'craziness'.

The soldier in this story was not trying to assault a child, but to make love to a young woman. While it is quite possible that a similar incident might happen in reality, we do not usually warn children about this kind of danger. A sixteen-year-old girl told me about a more common experience:

When I was about eight a man called me over to his car and he didn't have any trousers on and that came as such a shock — I never told anybody, I never told my mum — I think that's the only thing I never told her. 'Cos I didn't really understand, you know, I didn't think it was wrong or anything — I thought he'd get a cold sitting there without any trousers on, you know — it just didn't seem like anything.

This incident did not turn out to be dangerous. But the girl's failure to recognize it as sexual or to identify it as 'wrong' indicates that she would not have been very well prepared if it had become more serious.

The fears we have for children in circumstances like these are for their physical and psychological well-being. Even when they have not been physically injured we worry about the trauma they may suffer. Psychologists tend to stress the need for sensitive treatment for young victims, and warn that they are unlikely to develop a 'healthy' attitude to sexuality without this remedial action.

Neither in the fictional nor in the factual incidents I have just described did the girls seem to suffer any

61

mental damage, even when they realized later on what the experiences meant. Frankie is shaken and scared, but mainly because she thinks she might have killed the soldier and fears arrest and imprisonment. Her greater trauma is still to come with the shattering of her romantic dreams about her 'membership' of her brother's wedding, itself not unconnected with her sexual ignorance. The real-life experience obviously confused and disturbed the child, but as a young woman of sixteen she was able to discuss sex with ease and maturity, and described her current sexual relations as relaxed and fulfilling.

The reason why neither of these experiences caused psychological damage may well lie in a feature they have in common: neither girl told anyone what had happened. When early sexual encounters inflict no physical harm, most of the 'trauma' is probably caused by adult reaction. Children with no knowledge of sex are unlikely to attach the same significance to such encounters as adults would. If they can interpret an event only in terms of the shock of their elders it may be made to seem more terrifying than it actually was, and they may even feel guilt about it. A child who has been taught that the body is something private and forbidden may already feel uneasy and embarrassed about the incident, and if adults seem to be horrified more by its sexual content than by the force involved, these feelings are likely to be exacerbated. Rather than directing destructive emotions towards their attackers, children like this may turn them inwards against themselves and feel degraded or discredited. They may not be able to disentangle sex from these negative associations of disgust and self-denigration. Both adult and child victims of sexual attack may need support before they can come to terms with what has happened to them, yet the well-intentioned concern for child victims often adds to rather than allays their shock.

All this is in no way intended as an apology for child molestation. To be forced, persuaded or tricked into sexual intimacy against your will is to have your privacy invaded and your humanity denied. Without a doubt, any form of sexual coercion is reprehensible, and children who do not understand what is being done to them are being both coerced and exploited. It is difficult to imagine any sexual contact between a child and an adult where this would not be so, given adults' power over children and our readiness to use it to serve our own interests rather than theirs. Of course, this is true of many everyday activities, not just sexual ones, but for some reason it is not regarded as objectionable except in this context. The problem is not sex itself, but its association with power. In an ideal world, where coercion featured less in adult—child relationships and was altogether absent from sexual ones, the idea of imposing one's desires on someone smaller, weaker or less experienced would be unthinkable. For the time being, however, children have to make their way in a society where adults' power over them is inescapable and where aggression and sexuality are hopelessly entangled. If they are to succeed they need to know something of the lore of the sexual jungle.

A child who is aware of sexuality early in life will not fall victim to sexual exploitation through ignorance, but may well be vulnerable in other ways. Such a child, at home with her own sexuality, may find that her openness could be thought provocative by potential molesters and rapists. Moreover, if she has learnt to regard sex as a pleasurable experience creating mutual enjoyment, she will not be prepared for the possibility of anyone using it as a weapon against her. Children like her need to learn caution. Here is a predicament: how can we teach children to see sex positively, while at the same time warning them that it can be used to hurt and humiliate them?

The idea that an experience might be pleasurable in one context and not in another is probably not beyond the grasp of the average child. Children know, for example, that it is enjoyable to eat food they like when they are hungry, while being forced to eat something they dislike when they are not hungry is unpleasant and humiliating. They should be able to understand by analogy that sexual activity is enjoyable when it is desired and involves someone they like (including themselves), but unpleasant if they are forced into it when they do not feel like it or with someone they dislike. A small girl who is aware of her own body and knows about adult sexuality will also probably realize that intercourse with an adult man is likely to be painful. Children need to know too that some people would be prepared to use violence on them. They have to discover that the world is not all sweetness and light; they must learn that sexuality is no exception.

Children who are casual and uninhibited about sexuality also confront other more mundane problems, in particular the reactions of people who do not share their outlook. These children will at some point have to come to terms with conventional moral views and discover that behaviour which passes without comment in their immediate circle might provoke hostility from other adults. But again this is not a problem unique to sex. Children who grow up in a complex society like ours learn sooner or later that

64

the values and attitudes they have been taught at home are not shared by everyone. Children can cope with these differences of opinion in other areas, and I have known them cope with confrontations about their own sexual behaviour.

One example was when a friend of mine, Jean, took the five-year-old daughter of a friend with her on a visit to her parents. The child, whom I shall call Lynda (her own choice of alias), had been sexually aware from an early age and had developed an unself-conscious acceptance of her own and others' sexuality. At breakfast one morning she casually turned to Jean's mother and asked 'How do you masturbate?' Receiving no reply, she continued, 'I do it like this,' and proceeded to demonstrate. The question was probably as innocent as asking 'Do you like sugar?' to her, and she was unprepared for the shocked and angry response it provoked. Puzzled, she sat in silence through the heated argument that followed. The incident could have been a nasty shock for a girl who had never before been told that certain things were 'dirty' or 'disgusting', but she learnt a valuable lesson. She may have already guessed that anything to do with sex is taboo to some people, but had no real understanding of the implications until now. It is perhaps unfortunate that children have to be exposed to contradictory attitudes, but we can never shield them completely from the outside world, and the possibility that children might encounter clashes like this is hardly a good reason for keeping them ignorant. Lynda does not seem to have suffered any permanent damage as a result of her experience. Three years later she is still the same lively, bright and uninhibited child — though maybe a somewhat wiser one.

As I have tried to show, there seems to be no

justification for partitioning sex off from the rest of experience and concealing it from children. On the whole they would be better prepared to cope with the social world if this particular aspect of it was made known to them. Conventions that have been with us for centuries, however, are not so easily discarded; most of us observe them almost automatically. Most adults, even with the best of intentions, find it difficult to overcome their anxieties about children and sex and examine the strategies of concealment and secrecy that result from them. If we wish to bring about change and encourage more openness, how do we set about it? One thing we should try to avoid is a forced unselfconsciousness. If we do not ourselves have relaxed and positive attitudes to sexuality, it will not be easy for our children to acquire them. Indeed, parents who go out of their way to be open about sex despite feeling uncomfortable about it are likely to convey their uneasiness to their children.

If we are to allow children to accumulate sexual knowledge in the same way that they find out about other activities, they must be reared in an environment where information is available as a matter of course. Some of the children I know seem to have learnt about sex right from the beginning, acquiring their knowledge as easily and spontaneously as they learnt to walk and talk. I talked to the people who brought them up to try and find out how this was achieved. Their answers coincide with what I have noticed: sex was never hidden from the children, but neither was it deliberately forced on their attention. We do not need to invite children to watch us making love, but neither do we need to confine our sexual activities to times when they are not around, rapidly disentangling ourselves and evading questions if they discover us and ask what we are doing.

Children learn a great deal simply by listening to others' conversations and asking questions about what they hear. For example, in households where politics are frequently discussed, quite young children may show a surprising political awareness. This is not because someone has sat them down and lectured to them on socialism or fascism, but simply reflects a more general awareness of what is going on around them. If sexuality is openly discussed, a similar awareness will probably result.

Our attitudes to our own bodies may also teach children something about sexuality. When nakedness is accepted and children have the opportunity to observe the bodies of adults and children of both sexes, they will learn to name their own and others' genitals as easily as they learn to name fingers and toes. They will probably ask questions or make remarks about what they see, so drawing out further information and learning about both the sexual and the reproductive functions of various organs as easily as they learn that ears are for hearing and noses for smelling.

Unfortunately it is far easier to identify and criticize the obstacles to children's learning about sex than it is to recommend methods of overcoming them. The crucial factor seems to be the gulf we have created between sexual and non-sexual aspects of life, between sexual and other forms of relationship, between sexual organs and other parts of the body. In trying to close this gap, to make less of these distinctions, we may go some way towards creating conditions in which children can come to terms with sexuality more easily. Under such conditions, phrases like 'not in front of the children' or 'for adults only' would become obsolete.

5

Are Children Sexual?

Exactly what are we doing to children in keeping them ignorant of sex? The usual answer is deceptively simple: we are repressing their sexuality. People take this for granted when they discuss the ill effects of sexual taboos on children, particularly if they favour a more open attitude to sexuality. They tend to assume that the natural process of sexual development in childhood is being distorted by the repressive forces of our culture. In other words, they assume that children are naturally sexual: their sexuality would blossom and flourish of its own accord if only we would leave it alone. But would it? I think it is more likely that by keeping sex from children we are simply preventing them from becoming sexual — that is, delaying the development of sexual desires and behaviour that have to be learnt.

This may seem a strange claim, for it is customary to talk about sexuality in terms of inborn drives, urges that would be acted out in natural, spontaneous sexuality were they not held in check by outside influences. Even if it is accepted that culture moulds sexuality, it is often believed that a basic drive still exists which is the source of all our sexual needs and desires. But what would 'natural' sexuality, uncontaminated by cultural influences, be like? It is hard to imagine. If we do try to speculate, all we are doing is giving shape to our highest hopes or worst fears about sex. As we cannot determine what is natural and what not, surely it is better to suspend our curiosity about the unknowable and concentrate instead on how people become sexual in particular societies.

I want to suggest that when we look at children's experiences on the way to sexual maturity, what we see is a cumulative process of learning to become sexual and not the repression, channelling or moulding of existing sexual energies. We therefore need to be cautious about using such terms as 'infantile' and 'childhood' sexuality. If, as I have argued, the erotic significance of an act or situation lies in the meanings we apply to it, a child who has not yet learnt these meanings cannot be regarded as fully sexual.

This does not mean that children are incapable of experiencing sexual feelings and sensations or of engaging in sexual activities. But the ways in which we express our sexuality depend on how we interpret our feelings and desires and what we decide to do about them. We should not assume, when children do apparently sexual things, that they are motivated by the same wants and needs that we feel. Children may experience sensations similar to an adult's, but they are not usually able to make sense of them in the same way.

For example, anyone who can remember masturbating to orgasm as a child without knowing quite what they were doing will realize that the physical sensations they felt then are just the same as those they feel as adults. But it is doubtful if the act meant the same in childhood. As adults we can relate masturbation to other aspects of sexuality: we can draw on our sexual knowledge to construct elaborate fantasies that heighten our enjoyment, or can merely take pleasure in our ability to turn ourselves on. But this ability to make sense of masturbation in sexual terms is likely to be beyond the reach of a child. She or he knows that the activity is pleasurable and gratifying, but so are many other things. Masturbation may feel unique because of its climaxes and its ability to release tension, but it is still not prompted by the sexual arousal that an adult might feel.

It takes more than the simple act itself to grant masturbation any special meaning in the child's eyes. Perhaps adults' reactions have made it a covert activity, for instance. This need for secrecy may make the child feel guilty about masturbating, but even this emotion is different in kind from the guilt adults might feel. The child knows only that he or she is being naughty and might be punished if found out, but adults' guilt would be bound up with their feelings about sexuality in general. Children may link masturbation with other activities that draw similar responses from adults, such as taking off their clothes in front of other people (probably the nearest most get to finding material to furnish masturbatory fantasies), but they cannot experience sexual fantasies since they do not even know what sex is.

The danger here lies in reading too much into children's behaviour. We may remember sexual feelings and sensations associated with our own childhood activities, but this does not mean that we attached the same significance to them at the time, for in recalling our experiences we are reinterpreting them with the hindsight of adult knowledge. Similarly, when we observe a child's behaviour it is all too easy to grant it a meaning of which the child is unaware.

If sexuality amounted to nothing more than a series of physical sensations and patterns of behaviour, an outpouring of sexual energies, then it would be possible to argue that children are sexual. If, as I have been arguing, it is something more than this, something that must be understood in human and social terms, a sexually unaware child can only be described as *potentially* sexual, not actually so. It follows that there is no reason why children should not be sexual. Their sexuality lies not in a lack of capacity, but in a lack of opportunity; their inability to make sense of the world in sexual terms derives from ignorance, the result of the withholding of relevant information from them.

The claim that there is such a thing as childhood sexuality, that it exists independently of sexual knowledge, rests on a definition of sex as the development of inbuilt drives through predetermined states, ending with mature, adult sexuality. This is a perspective associated with the Freudian psychoanalytic tradition. It is worth looking a little more closely at it, for it has influenced much modern thinking on children and sex, and the basic assumptions behind it are accepted by many people who would not count themselves as Freudians. This perspective has also found its way into many popular works and has been incorporated into textbooks for trainee teachers, nurses and social workers, child-rearing manuals for parents and sex education books for young people.

It is not my intention to enter into a detailed analysis of Freud's work or to make any contribution to the innumerable (and often tedious) academic

71

debates about what he really said, really meant or really meant to say. Instead I will concentrate on those ideas which have filtered through to everyday knowledge. Since this popularized version of Freud is based upon a literal understanding of his work that assumes that he said exactly what he meant and meant exactly what he said, my comments will also be based upon that assumption.

The Freudian tradition traces the development of the libido through a series of changes that are thought to condition the final, mature form of human sexuality. Sexual experiences in childhood are supposed to affect not only the individual's sexual life but the whole human personality, and especially those attributes we associate with femininity and masculinity. The path of development is said to be predetermined by nature, though it is realized through our participation in social institutions such as the family.

This perspective depends upon classifying a wide range of infant and childhood behaviour as sexual, as involving the same basic needs as adult sexuality. Almost everything in which a child finds sensual pleasure is labelled sexual, as are emotional attachments, especially with parents.

It is indeed likely that the kinds of physical sensation we learn to enjoy as children will affect our adult sexuality, as will the ways we have found of expressing and controlling our emotions. But I would argue that this hardly makes them sexual in some absolute and undeniable sense, and it certainly does not make them an inevitable part of development. The mistake here is in classifying behaviour according to its external character rather than in terms of its subjective meaning. It is quite possible, using the former strategy, to lump together every kind of sensual

72

pleasure, but it is misleading to call them all sexual. I might gain sensual pleasure from stoking a cat, eating good Italian food or being in bed with a lover, but these activities in no way mean the same thing to me, nor are they inspired by similar needs. Freudians are apt to link quite disparate experiences together along these lines so that a child's enjoyment of thumb-sucking, playing on swings, riding on trains or sitting on horseback are all seen as sexual, gratifying the same needs. It is surely more logical, though, to view sex as one form of pleasure rather than all pleasure as sexual. This latter option simply does not make sense if we judge our feelings and actions — as we usually do from day to day — by the significance they have for us.

The problem with any criticism of this type of psychoanalysis is that people who accept its basic propositions tend to embrace the conclusions that follow with an unshakeable faith. Almost any appeal to the way we actually experience things in everyday life can be met with the rebuff 'Ah, but sub-consciously . . .'. For anyone with this belief in the subconscious it is an easy matter to impose a fixed set of ideas onto someone's experience and then claim to have explained it.

One experience considered crucial within Freudian theory, penis envy, will serve to illustrate some of the problems attached to this system of thought. When a small girl, perhaps three years old, first sets eyes on the male sexual organ she is supposed to be overcome by an intense envy, a realization that her puny clitoris cannot match the mighty penis, that it is less suitable for masturbation and altogether inferior. The desire to possess an appendage as wonderful as the male's is said to mark her for life, to be the single most important influence on her sexuality. But how do little girls really react when they discover this difference between the sexes?

In the first place, there seems no obvious reason why a small girl should admire or covet a penis. If she feels her own body to be whole and complete, it is more likely that she will, on first seeing a male one, regard it as a deformed rather than improved version. This is indeed a very common reaction. I well remember my younger sister's discovery of this difference when she was at about the age when penis envy is supposed to occur. On a visit to our local shop we saw a woman carrying a naked small boy. My sister stared hard at him, an expression of total disgust on her face, then pointed and said, very loudly, 'Ugh! That little boy's got a horrible thing growing out of his bottom!' Was she really sublimating her envy, covering up some deep sense of personal inadequacy? It seems to me that her reaction was quite spontaneous and honest, and did not mask any brooding feeling of failure lurking in the subconscious.

I cannot recall when I first noticed that boys' bodies were different from mine, but I do remember some of my thoughts later when I was about seven or eight. At that time I viewed male genitals with a mixture of fascination and revulsion, much the same as I might have felt about physical deformity. I also reflected about the possibility of male masturbation. I masturbated at the time and assumed that other people must do so too. I concluded, however, that it must be an entirely female activity — boys would find it difficult because their 'thing' would get in the way. If there is little reason to assume that a small girl sees a penis as a desirable asset, there is still less reason why she should think it is anything other than a

74

urinary organ. She need not know that she has a clitoris in order to masturbate effectively, and even if she does, will she necessarily see it as a miniature penis, or make the next step and conclude that bigger must be better?

There are children who fit the Freudian model rather better; they discover the penis at the appropriate age and do display some signs of envy. Here is a conversation between two three-year-olds, a boy and a girl:

Girl: Are you playing with your penis?
Boy: Yes. Are you playing with your vagina?
Girl: Yes. [Looking at boy's penis and picking up a toy dagger.]
I'm going to cut it off and try it on me.

The little girl clearly expresses the desire to own a penis, but how important is it to her? The conversation was quite a casual one and the children soon passed on to other amusements, neither giving the impression of having suffered any trauma. The girl announced her wish to try on the boy's penis in much the same tone as she would have used had the object of her 'envy' been a hat or a tee shirt. There seems little basis for deducing that the girl has begun to suffer from a deep-seated feeling of deprivation that will remain with her for life. And what, with castration fears figuring so large in Freudian theory, did the boy make of all this? Apparently little: he seemed not at all worried by the playful threat and like the girl soon turned his attention to other matters.

Another common childhood experience that Freudians overemphasize is the feeling that one's genitals might change. It is usually interpreted as a fear of castration in boys and as masculine striving brought on by penis envy in girls, and both are supposed to leave indelible marks on the child's psyche. But small children, looking at their own and other people's bodies, often do not realize that they are endowed with one particular set of genitals for life, or that this is what defines them as female or male. After all, the body of an adult of the same sex may look as different from their own as that of a child of the opposite sex, as long as the presence or absence of a penis is not taken as the only point of comparison. There is no reason why children should not believe that their sex organs, like other things, might change as they grow older. I have known small boys, fascinated by women's breasts, ask if they will grow some one day or express the hope that they might. Is this any different from a girl thinking she might grow a penis? Do boys suffer from 'breast envy'? Moreover, children tend to determine the sex of their friends by, say, dress or hair length rather than by their genitals; indeed they often think these are quite irrelevant. The little boy mentioned earlier happens to have rather beautiful long hair. Once when several children were playing together unclothed, his mother overheard another child saying of him 'That little girl's got a penis.' A story sent to a magazine further illustrates the point. A small girl announced that she had been swimming naked with some other children. 'Were they boys or girls?' she was asked. 'I don't know,' she replied, 'they didn't have any clothes on.'

Many children, either because of prudish upbringing or because of the lack of brothers or sisters, do not discover that girls and boys have different sex organs until they are way past the age when genital traumas are supposed to take effect. Are we to believe that girls in this position somehow subconsciously suffer penis envy even when they have never seen one? This would seem rather far-fetched.

All this suggests that it is dangerous to infer too much from children's interest in their own and others' genitals — it might have nothing to do with sexual desires and have little effect on later sexual development. Of course, I cannot hope to challenge a firmly rooted belief in penis envy; almost anything can be attributed to the subconscious, and anything I have said can be twisted to fit the theory. But there is nothing that would serve as definite proof that penis envy exists. Freud himself said that if the concept was dismissed as an 'idée fixe' then he was 'defenceless', suggesting that he was powerless to defend a major pillar of his theory. The only way in which penis envy makes sense is as a general envy of maleness, with the penis taken as a symbol of it. But if this is so it can hardly be associated so closely with children's discoveries about genitals or regarded as such a major force in sexual development.

So the basic faults in the psychoanalytic approach lie in overestimating children's sexual capacities and attaching too much sexual significance to their desires and activities. These traps are easy to fall into if we interpret children's actions through the filter of adult sexual knowledge and experience. To avoid it we need to question how far children's behaviour can be seen as sexual (that is, as sexually motivated and meaningful) and this means that we should look closely at the desires and interests we attribute to them.

Despite the great influence of the psychoanalytic tradition on our everyday attitudes to children and sex, our reactions to manifestations of 'childhood sexuality' are more complex and contradictory. Often Freudian ideas have had more effect on the aspects of child-rearing that we do not generally regard as sexual, such as toilet training, than on those where sexuality is directly concerned. The relatively recent contribution of psychoanalysis is still largely overshadowed by earlier ideas, hopes and fears about children and sex. Though childhood sexuality may be given undue emphasis in some textbooks and child-care manuals, many adults today still find it difficult to confront the possibility that children might be sexual.

The psychologist Leah Cahan Schaefer has observed that adults either overestimate or underestimate children's sexual capacities. It is my belief that we frequently do both. The image of children as asexual innocents is still with us, implying that children lack sexual interests and desires and cannot cope with sexual knowledge. Yet the steps we take in order to preserve this innocence suggest there is some uncertainty, that we fear children are not as innocent as we might wish. The conflicting images of the innocent and demoniac child continue to pull us both ways. Hence the paradox that even while underestimating children's sexual potential we overestimate it; even while we insist that children must be 'protected' from sex we treat anything they do or say that seems sexual as if it were motivated by fully-formed sexual interests. Thus, while preventing children from becoming sexually aware, adults often respond to them as if they already were. It seems there is a great deal of confusion about whether children are sexual and if so, in what sense. Such inconsistencies and contradictions in our attitudes must be ironed out if we are ever to understand what happens in the course of a child's sexual development.

The question of whether children have the physical potential to be sexual is easily answered: they do. The capacity for arousal and orgasm is present from birth. If the arguments I presented in chapter 4 are accepted, there appears to be no reason to suppose that children lack the mental capacity to make sense of sexuality. In other words, children could be sexual if we did not discourage the development of their physical capacities and deny them access to information which would allow them to understand their own and others' experience in sexual terms. Children who are prevented from acquiring sexual awareness are *not* fully sexual beings.

The aspect of early development which has the greatest impact on our sexuality is not specifically sexual. It is through learning about gender — discovering the significance accorded to the differences between the sexes, and developing a sense of themselves as feminine or masculine — that children begin to develop a basis for later sexual learning. Girls and boys learn to be sexual in different ways and it is in childhood, when they begin to learn to think and act in accordance with our ideals of femininity and masculinity, that the foundations of these different styles of sexuality are built. Children's understanding of gender will affect the ways they react to sexual information and link it to their own feelings and experiences. Young people in our society learn about sex as heterosexuality, the relationships between women and men, so it is only to be expected that they associate it with what they already know about gender. Such continuity as there is between childhood and adolescence consists chiefly of the images of ourselves and others as feminine or masculine; through them we make sense of the sexual world and place ourselves within it.

All the same, some childhood experiences do contribute to a young person's understanding of sex once they have been fused with new knowledge. These are those incidents that the child does not see as sexual at the time, but that may be open to re-interpretation once the basic sexual facts are known. Memories of 'sexual' games, of curiosity about our bodies, of certain feelings and experiences, may all be counted as sexual when we look back on them. This does not mean that childhood experiences prior to sexual awareness in any way determine later, conscious sexual learning. They simply provide an adolescent with some personal memories that might take on new meaning when reconsidered in the light of new sexual knowledge, and thus contribute to the formation of ideas about sexuality.

At this point in sexual development, the present restructures the past as much as the past influences the present. The childhood experiences were not sexual at the time, but only become so through re-interpretation. This type of learning, which might be called 'protosexual', is very different from that involved in the learning of gender and has less far-reaching consequences for later sexual development, as I shall explain in chapter 6. A child is able to amass a reasonably integrated body of knowledge about gender, building up a picture of what it means to be male or female and where s/he fits in. Protosexual learning, on the other hand, generally consists of isolated or arbitrary incidents that may, when placed in the context of sexual knowledge later on, have some sexual significance. These fragments have little meaning for young children. From their point of view the sexual world is like a giant jigsaw puzzle. They have access to a few of the pieces, but most have been hidden from them, so they have no way of knowing how the pieces fit together or even that they belong to the same puzzle. Only when the missing pieces are supplied, when the pieces begin to fit and the puzzle begins to take shape, can children make any real sense of sexuality and interpret and act on their sexual feelings.

So children are neither naturally sexual nor naturally asexual. But if we are preventing children from becoming sexual by keeping them ignorant of sex, we cannot assume that we do no damage to them in the process. To dispense with ideas about sexual drives and repression is not to absolve ourselves of guilt or responsibility; we still cannot afford to disregard young people's problems as they try to come to terms with sexuality. I have already suggested that in keeping children sexually ignorant we may expose them to danger and anxiety. We also make their sexual learning more troublesome, confusing and upsetting than it need be.

6

The Dark Age:
Children and Sexual Learning

The early years of childhood may not be a period of conscious sexual learning, but they cannot be dismissed as irrelevant to the process of sexual development. Although the emergence of sexuality is delayed until adolescence, it is in childhood that its foundations are laid down.

I have identified two types of learning which contribute to this process: the development of gender identity, which serves as a focus of later sexual learning, and 'protosexual' experiences, which may teach children something about the conventions and morality of adult sex when they are able to reinterpret them later in the light of sexual awareness. These two processes are quite distinct from each other, converging only when they are integrated into a body of knowledge, when they will each contribute to sexual development in their different ways. Both deserve closer scrutiny.

So far I have talked about children in general, making little distinction between boys and girls. What all children share — their status as a special category of people, the sexual ignorance that is but one sign of their exclusion from adult life — is ultimately overshadowed by the fact that they are born into a society bisected by gender. The first comment that greets an infant emerging into the world is usually: 'It's a girl' or 'It's a boy'. From that point on the child will be expected to become feminine or masculine and in so doing she or he will develop a basis for the specific forms of sexual expression typical of women and men in our society.

Gender and sexuality are inextricably linked. Sexual learning is part of gender learning, for we learn to be sexual as women or as men. We learn also that we are expected to direct our sexual interest towards the opposite sex, and that in our sexual relations we are supposed to bridge the gap created by gender. Even if we reject heterosexuality, our sexual lives are organized around the existence of gender.

Gender is the single most important aspect of our personal identity. We cannot think of ourselves without being aware that we are female or male, nor relate to others without attaching the appropriate gender labels to them. The first thing we notice about anyone we meet, as with the new-born baby, is their sex. We feel uncomfortable in the presence of someone whose sex is uncertain, for we rely on the help of stereotypes to tell us what to expect from women and men. We take it for granted that others are aware of our own sex and behave towards us accordingly, even if we resent it. Try to imagine what people would be like in a world without gender, or read Ursula le Guin's *The Left Hand of Darkness*, in which a visitor to Gethen, a planet inhabited by hermaphrodites, comments: 'One is respected and judged only as a human being. It is an appalling experience.' All our lives we are judged as women or as men, hardly ever just as human beings. Our language forces us to think in terms of she and he and our culture teaches us to think of them as quite separate categories. The distinctions we make between masculine and feminine are as great as those we draw between childhood and adulthood, but whereas the status of child is a temporary one, gender is permanent and inescapable.

Learning about gender is not just a process whereby we come to think of ourselves as female or male, it affects all aspects of our personality and involves more than learning labels and the patterns of behaviour that go with them. Attitudes and emotions, character traits, aptitudes, ambitions and desires are all bound up with gender and learnt as part of our 'gender role'.

I am not saying that sheer indoctrination is what makes children learn to think, feel and act in terms of gender; the process is much more subtle and complex than that. It is not just a question of playing with dolls and train sets or being influenced by parents and teachers. The process of gender learning has been the subject of much research and theorizing that I cannot summarize in detail here. Instead I shall give a broad outline and isolate those factors that seem to have the greatest effect on sexuality.

A child's induction into our gender-divided world begins at the very moment of birth, when a whole range of expectations come into play and mental pictures are formed of the sort of person the baby will become. Even the new-born are stereotyped by gender; for example, baby girls are immediately described as 'sweet' or 'pretty', while most parents would be grossly offended to hear these words applied to their baby son; the only creature I've ever heard called 'pretty boy' was a parrot. For boys the comments are different: 'Isn't he active!' or 'You can see he's going to be strong' or 'He's a proper little man'. If people impose ideas like these on infants whose sex cannot even be distinguished, it is hardly surprising that girls and boys are treated quite differently from very early in their lives. A self-fulfilling prophesy begins to unfold: babies are treated as if they already were feminine or masculine, and so, in the course of time, they become feminine or masculine. Some of the differences of treatment result from quite conscious decisions, such as the choice of names and clothes for babies; others are unintentional, expressed through the ways we talk to, handle and play with them. Adults are often unaware that they are making these distinctions, and in any case we take it for granted that girls and boys will behave differently, enjoy different things and want different toys, so they are treated accordingly. Throughout childhood they will learn that what is expected of them depends on their gender.

The effects of this learning begin to show very early. If by some accident a child is wrongly sexed at birth, perhaps because there is a genital abnormality, by the time it is two it will be difficult to correct the faulty labelling, and by five it will be virtually impossible. The results of early learning are so indelible that one cannot then convince a child of its 'real' sex. Children grow up to possess the characteristics of the gender they are assigned to, not their biological sex. It is quite possible for a child to grow up into an adult whose gender conflicts with his or her biological sex. Work carried out with such children has taught us a great deal about how gender identity is established.

By the time children are two or three they know their own sex, and over the next few years they learn to label others correctly. Once they reach five or six they are aware that they will remain the same sex for life, girls becoming women and boys becoming men. It is then that gender identity is totally fixed and becomes central to children's images of themselves.

Children of this age will have come to match our ideas of what little girls and little boys should be like. They will have acquired ways of thinking and feeling and behaving that our society considers distinctly feminine or masculine. Children learn these things easily. Being wholly dependent on the care and affection of the adults around them, they will do their best to respond to any demands so as to gain approval. In their earliest years they know only that certain behaviour is judged good or bad, but once they have learnt their gender role they begin to anticipate what is required of them and will act in an appropriate way without the help of direct instruction. They will gravitate towards activities that fit their awareness of their sex, since this now helps them maintain a positive image of themselves. For example, investigation of children's play shows that they will be more interested in a particular toy or game if they think it is suitable for their sex than if they see it as more fitting for the opposite sex, or as something either boys or girls can use. Children have plenty of sources from which to draw conclusions about what is feminine or masculine. Books, toys, television programmes and their experience of the adult world all serve to inform them about their proper role. They are also able to identify with adults of the same sex, and are often encouraged to do so, with phrases like 'just like Mummy' or 'just like Daddy' uttered in approving tones.

Girls often find this indentification easier than boys, since our society so organizes child-care and schooling that younger children come far more in contact with women than with men. Boys seem to acquire masculine characteristics as much by avoiding anything feminine as by imitating men directly: the models most available to them are not men they actually know, but fantasy figures from television screens and comics. This pattern carries over to children's toys and games: girls' activities bear a much greater resemblance to those of the average woman than boys' do to the average man's. Girls may play at housewives, mothers or nurses, but whoever heard of small boys playing assembly-line workers or insurance salesmen? Two things are happening here. Firstly, girls are learning that their world is relatively limited, and boys that theirs holds endless possibilities. Secondly, while boys or girls may affect disdain for the other sex, boys generally express it much more strongly, thus learning to denigrate all things female — an attitude which may stay with them for life. These messages about gender are so far-reaching that they even affect children who are brought up in households that try to counteract such stereotypes. I have known many feminists whose young sons have told them that women are not allowed or are too stupid to do something or other. My own sister, brought up by a working mother and an ambitious elder sister both of whom tried to steer her clear of the worst types of femininity, still assumed as a small child that most of the world's occupations and pastimes were closed to women.

So children are not only learning to be feminine or masculine but also discovering that one is not valued as highly as the other. A result of this can perhaps be seen in a phenomenon that has puzzled psychologists and sociologists for some time: girls between the ages of five and ten seem much more reluctant to accept their role than boys of the same age do. Two possible interpretations have been offered. One is that children are aware that men hold more prestigious positions than women in our society, so while boys are eager to grasp all the opportunities their sex affords them, girls try to avoid the shackles of femininity for as long as they can. Alternatively, it may be that those 'unfeminine' qualities and actions observed in girls do not indicate a rebellion against femininity; perhaps they can reconcile a degree of tomboyishness with more traditionally feminine attitudes. Boys may avoid girls' activities more than the reverse because boys tend to establish their gender by avoiding all things feminine; or the answer may simply be that to be a tomboy is socially acceptable, even approved of, while to be a cissy most certainly is not. So girls often play quite happily with both boys' and girls' toys, while boys are usually horrified at the idea of venturing beyond the strict confines of masculinity: the average small boy will be outraged if you call his Action Man a doll.

Whatever the reasons for these differences, most girls as well as boys do adapt to the role they have been allotted. Children have to fit into the world as they see it, for they are not experienced enough to know how to rebel.

This, then, is the pattern of gender-learning in childhood. But what has it all got to do with sexuality?

In the first place, these feminine and masculine attributes will be incorporated later in life into sexual activities and relationships. Because boys are encouraged to be independent and exercise their own judgement, while girls are expected to be dependent and compliant, it is not surprising that men usually take the initiative in sexual relationships. Because boys learn dominance, girls submission, the most common position for sex has the man on top, the woman supine beneath him in symbolic affirmation of their relative social status. Because boys learn to be physically aggressive, as men they are capable of using sex as a means of coercion; if they have learnt to regard women as inferiors, the likelihood becomes that much greater. Because girls' emotional capacities are developed to a greater extent, their sexuality will be more closely tied up with feeling and they will find it harder to divorce sex and affection. Because boys have a choice of how to prove their masculinity, while girls' opportunities to affirm their femininity are more limited, girls come to regard long-term, romantic relationships as more central to their lives, and so invest more in them.

I could give many more illustrations of this kind to prove the same point: that becoming feminine means preserving certain child-like qualities, while becoming masculine means growing away from them. Characteristics that would seem ridiculous in men are thought sexually attractive in women. For instance, we are apt to think of children as cute, and they learn to play on this to manipulate adults and gain approval. At some point, however, boys discover that they are considered too old for this game and that it no longer works for them, whereas it goes on working for girls — 'playing cute' is a strategy many young women use to attract men. Vulnerability is also valued in women, and certain female fashions, such as totally impractical shoes and flimsy dresses, serve to accentuate it. Many of the conventions of heterosexual relationships emphasize that the man is 'looking after' the women. He must appear to make the decisions: ordering food in restaurants, buying tickets for the theatre or cinema, adopting protective poses.

In sexual relationships it is the man who is expected to be active, the woman merely attractive, and again this is a pattern established in childhood. Since the emergence of the woman's movement the idea that women are sexual objects has become a cliché. But while clichés inevitably distort reality, they generally reflect some basic truth too, and the role of sexual object is one that little girls begin to learn very early in life. While boys learn that social approval is earned by what they do, girls learn that it derives from what they are. They are discouraged from acting independently and encouraged to be pliant, to please others, to be dependent on others' opinions rather than their own judgement. Anyone who has ever heard parents or teachers of young children comparing boys and girls may have noticed the approval boyish disobedience and stubbornness often secures. Provided it is not too extreme, it is regarded as a sign of masculinity and greeted with a smile or shrug — 'Boys will be boys.' The same behaviour in a girl, however, provokes frowns and worried tones and is thought a real problem. Teachers are apt to attibute girls' early educational success to their neatness, lack of restlessness and eagerness to please, qualities boys lack, making them much less easy to teach.

As well as acquiring this passivity, girls also learn the importance of being pretty, a major way of gaining the approval on which they are beginning to depend. From the first time someone coos over her cot and tells her how sweet she looks, a girl is encouraged to cultivate physical attractiveness. Fussy, frilly clothes are no longer fashionable for small girls, but they still tend to be dressed in less functional garments than boys, ones that incorporate purely decorative features and are more easily damaged. Wearing them not only emphasizes girls' passive prettiness, but also — because of the carefulness they demand of the wearer — encourages the dainty posture and demeanour so important to feminine physical attractiveness. Girls might be allowed to play in jeans and dungarees, but they still tend to be dressed up for special occasions.

When so arrayed girls are told how wonderful they look and made to feel that they have achieved something. They develop an interest in clothes and fashion early and will spend hours dressing up. Even the most confirmed tomboy often has a weakness for pretty things; in *The Member of the Wedding* Frankie is careless of her appearance most of the time, but insists on her best dress being perfectly pressed and buys an extravagant outfit for her brother's wedding. Most girls soon become self-conscious about their looks and acutely aware of how they compare (and compete) with others'. I can remember feeling a desperate envy for the golden curls some of my classmates had, hating my own dark, straight hair, not at all fashionable in the fifties. I longed for a party dress prettier than anyone else's and was delighted when my father bought me one made of yellow imitation silk, covered with cream lace and trimmed with tiny pink buttons. There is a photograph of me in this appalling garment at a party: I am holding out my full skirts and have an amazingly self-satisfied smirk on my face, knowing, for once, that my dress was the best.

Blessed is the pretty girl, conscious of her advantage, self-confident and popular. She hears adults comment on the less fortunate: 'Isn't it a pity she's not pretty.'

The plain girl's lot is not a happy one. Not long ago I watched a girl at a children's party. She was overweight, clumsy and, unlike the others, had no pretty clothes. She had been invited, much against the wishes of her little hostess, because she was a neighbour. It would have been kinder not to have bothered. None of the other girls talked to her; they made it clear they resented her presence, refused to partner her in games, and tried to avoid sitting next to her at the tea table. No little girl wants to be guilty, even by association, of not being pretty. They all learn that it is a means to success, and they may realize that the goal of adult womanhood, marriage, is thought to depend on it.

Boys are rarely made so self-conscious about their appearance. Unless they are grossly fat or wear bizarre clothes they are unlikely to be taunted about their looks. They may be expected to look smart on special occasions, but usually adults do not bother to fuss over their appearance or encourage them to be too concerned about it. I am willing to bet that few men can recall, as I and many other women can, precisely what they and their friends wore at parties: it simply wouldn't have been that important to them. Boys do not have to suffer all the restrictions imposed on little girls in the pursuit of prettiness — orders to 'sit up straight', 'smile' and so on. Later in their lives they may admire the results of girls' long beauty training, but as children they scorn it as just one more example of female silliness.

While girls learn the virtues of prettiness, boys are living far more boisterous, active lives. Their image of their physical selves rests on what their bodies can do, not what they look like. Boys learn to be rougher and tougher: they may be kissed and cuddled when very small, but not later on, when 'babying' them is frowned upon. Recently I saw a man refuse a kiss from a two-year-old boy. 'You're too old for that now,' he said, 'it's not manly.' But even when boys are young, adults, particularly men, will play rough-and-tumble games with them, so that they learn to associate affection and approval with a hearty slap on the back rather than a tender caress. Girls are exposed to more gentle physical contacts as examples of warmth and affection. Adults will continue to kiss and fondle them long after they have given up with boys. Girls come to see this behaviour as an integral part of any loving relationship and will expect it in later sexual experiences; boys will take some time to develop the necessary techniques, since their lack of experience of gentleness produces a more aggressive style of sexual expression. Many men find it difficult to show affection physically except through sex, and women who realize this sometimes engage in sex simply to receive affection. As a sixteen-year-old un-married mother told me, 'I didn't like the sex much — I did it for the cuddling-up afterwards.'

All the attitudes, feelings and responses that girls and boys learn come together in their ideas about the one aspect of adult sexual relationships they are allowed to witness as children: romanticism. Although they know little about sex, they are aware that certain adult relationships are special, different from mere friendship, involving something called 'love' and usually expected to culminate in marriage. Both girls and boys have this awareness, but they view the relationships quite differently.

Girls receive a thorough schooling in romanticism from their earliest years. They learn that winning the love of a man is a major achievement, the reward for

93

femininity. They learn that romance is wonderful; they see adult women read about it and gush over weddings. Weddings especially attract them: the whole idea of a dramatic spectacle with the beautifully-clad bride the centre of attention. As small girls they play at weddings and often long to be bridesmaids. They learn that this is the 'best day in a woman's life' — a phrase that was used time and time again when I talked to teenage girls. These girls, old enough not to have childish fantasies, had few opinions on marriage but knew what sort of wedding they wanted. Some had already planned it right down to the smallest detail, and were simply waiting for an appropriate groom to arrive and step into his appointed place. Many other aspects of romance appeal to small girls, since it incorporates all the qualities they have been trained in: pleasing others, being gentle and affection-ate, enjoying intense emotional relationships. Even tomboys find it hard to ignore romance and it is frequently the lure that will later draw them back towards more conventional feminine interests.

For boys the situation is very different. for if romance fits in precisely with feminine ideals it almost by definition clashes with masculine ones. Boys often seem to be embarrassed that adult men are implicated in it at all, for it is virtually the anti-thesis of everything they have been taught to consider manly. Small boys watching films or television will often be disgusted or lose interest if a love scene interrupts the more exciting action. As yet, ignorant of the sexual payoff, they have no way of knowing that this is just one more field for masculine prowess. All that a young boy sees in love and romance is qualities he has come to identify with females and learnt to despise. Romance, from his point of view, is incomprehensible, trivial, boring, definitely cissy and plain silly. It is beneath the dignity of any self-respecting male — and for that matter of any woman he sets above the common herd.

These attitudes and feelings are brought vividly to life in L.P. Hartley's novel *The Go-Between*. Leo, the young hero, fully supports the view that love is despicable. However, he has been carrying letters between Marian, the lady of the house where he is staying, and Ted, her humble-born lover. Entrusted with this task and sworn to secrecy, he imagines he is part of some mysterious, exciting adventure, perhaps even a matter of life and death. On one occasion Marian leaves an envelope unsealed; overcome by curiosity, Leo reads the letter and is shattered by the contents:

I felt utterly deflated and let down: so deep did my disappointment and disillusion go that I lost all sense of where I was and when I came to it was like waking from a dream.

They were in love! Marian and Ted Burgess were in love. Of all the possible explanations, it was the only one that had never crossed my mind. What a sell, what a frightful sell! And what a fool I had been! Trying to regain my self-respect, I allowed myself a hollow chuckle. To think how I had been taken in! . . . My only defence was that I could not have expected it of Marian . . . how could she have sunk so low? To be what we all despised more than anything — soft, soppy — hardly, when the joke grew staler, a subject for furtive giggling.

. . . I laughed and laughed . . . and at the same time [felt] miserable about it and obscurely aware that ridicule, however enjoyable, is no substitute for worship. That Marian of all people should have done this. No wonder she wanted it kept secret. Instinctively, to cover her shame, I thrust the letter deep into the envelope and sealed it.

The reaction of this Edwardian boy captures a feeling about romance that is still prevalent among sexually unaware boys today. Often the idea that love and romance is degrading stays with them through adolescence. When they find out about sex many are wary of linking it with romance, and even those who do become more romantically minded later in adolescence find it difficult to reconcile the two. Girls, on the other hand, tend to come to terms with sexuality only by associating it with love. Hence the seeds of later tensions and misunderstandings between lovers are sown in childhood.

An irony I have already noted is that in attempting to preserve children's innocence we may teach them about guilt. A major cause of guilt is adults' tendency to overestimate children's sexual capacities. Some of us can remember being caught while playing 'doctors and nurses', and the shocked, embarrassed or angry adult response that followed. Children in this situation are being judged by adults' sexual values without knowing what they are. All they know is that their actions have been called wrong or 'dirty', so they learn that they can only repeat them in secret and at risk of punishment. Thus children may begin to feel guilty and anxious about certain activities before they understand their sexual significance. Later, when the sexual undertones are apparent, this sense of furtiveness may become part of a young person's feelings about sexuality.

It may be that adults' reactions to children's

behaviour turn previously innocent activities into guilt-ridden ones, but many children will already have an inkling that 'sexual' games are taboo, infringing as they do the rules of modesty that have most likely already been learnt. Children are taught early on that certain parts of the body must be kept hidden and that it is 'rude' or 'dirty' to expose them to others. Their attitudes to their own genitals and feelings about bodily modesty are almost bound to affect the way they later come to terms with sexuality. The discovery of a new genital function — sex — will probably be interpreted in the light of what they have already learnt to think and feel about their bodies. Girls and boys are likely to see things differently, for girls tend to encounter more rigid restrictions than boys, thanks to our prevailing ideas about hygiene, modesty and sexuality. On the whole girls will be less ready to face the facts of sexuality and less likely to discover their genitals as a source of sexual pleasure.

During childhood, anatomy and social attitudes will combine to ensure that while boys at least become familiar with their sexual organs, girls may not even know that they have any. While children of either sex are likely to be firmly discouraged from masturbating, a boy cannot help but be aware of his penis, being expected to handle it when he urinates. A girl's genitals, on the other hand, are not so obvious, and she has no legitimate excuse to get familiar with that part of her body. Usually she will be told that to touch herself there is dirty, an idea that then becomes attached to her genitals and their secretions. The prohibition carries all the more weight because small girls are rigorously trained in the virtues of cleanliness. Small boys are often proud of their control of urination, happily showing off to their friends and competing with them in games, but girls learn to hide such shameful things behind locked doors.

If a small girls is to discover her hidden organs at all she must actively explore her body, which may be difficult as adults tend to object more to girls' genital play than boys'. The myth that men have a stronger sex drive means that though boys' masturbation may be seen as regrettable, it is at least understood and so is easier to tolerate. A typical mother's attitude is quoted by Pat Whiting in her study of female sexuality:

> I mean for *boys* it's only natural, they can't help themselves, but I wouldn't like to see my little girls touching herself. What would people think?

So it is that many girls know nothing about their sexual organs. I can remember, when I was thirteen, discussing with friends the problems of using tampons. Even supposing we could bring ourselves to touch ourselves 'down there', how were we to find our vaginas and be sure that we had located the right place? At least we all knew that we had a vagina. None of us had the slightest idea that we also had a clitoris.

There are other areas where adult notions of sexual propriety impinge on girls' lives. Sexual modesty is considered a specifically feminine virtue, so any signs of immodesty in girls are condemned most forcefully. In fact, girls are often so well schooled that they are even reluctant to reveal their bodies to other girls. To some the experience of communal school showers and shared changing rooms can be quite upsetting, even before the onset of puberty and physical development begin to cause embarrassment to both sexes. These problems are intensified by girls' clothing:

if we teach children that it is indecent to reveal their underwear, and then proceed to dress half of them in skirts, we are placing that half at a distinct disadvantage. Girls have to learn to avoid certain postures and exercises. They are told off for performing handstands and cartwheels if not properly dressed for gymnastics, for sitting cross-legged on the floor or with their knees apart, and for letting their skirts ride up. Many of the teenage girls I talked to had been given these warnings and found that they tended to be all the more strict as they approached puberty. Most women and girls in our society have probably had similar experiences.

Keeping these laws of sexual modesty is associated with the finer points of femininity. Girls are told that it is not only indecent to sit improperly, but also unattractive. As a result they may later find conventional sexual postures not merely immodest but also unfeminine, ugly and clumsy.

Girls also suffer greater disadvantages than boys because larger areas of their bodies are tabooed. Growing up in a society where female breasts are a sexual fetish, they must sooner or later learn that they too must be kept covered. They are usually expected to begin this concealment well before puberty, when their nipples are still indistinguishable from boys'. One girl told me:

> We used to live in a hot climate and I used to go round in my knickers without anything else on. But I was only, what, nine or ten, so it didn't matter, but my mother used to tell me off.

If her experience sounds unusual or her mother ridiculously puritanical, think what children usually

99

wear on the beach. Even the smallest girls are often dressed in tiny bikinis or one-piece swimsuits designed to cover the breast area.

As we have seen, little girls are likely to develop far more anxieties about their bodies than boys do, so that it is more difficult for them to accept sexuality later. These problems have often been taken to prove that girls are more sexually repressed, but it is not a case of repression, rather the learning of attitudes that will affect their feelings about sex, such as distaste and shame about normal bodily functions. Such attitudes may prevent the dawning of sexual awareness even when certain of the facts are within children's reach. Frankie in *The Member of the Wedding* again provides an example. Here she is reacting to something she has been told by older girls:

> They were talking nasty lies about married people. When I think of Aunt Pet and Uncle Eustace. And my own father! The nasty lies! I don't know what kind of fool they take me for.

Her response does not prove that a child cannot cope with sexual knowledge, but is rather the result of the concealment of sex coupled with the teaching that behaviour like this is inconceivable. Children are hardly likely to believe that adults they respect could engage in acts that combine the immodesty of nakedness, the adoption of ungainly postures, the touching of forbidden areas of the body and the dirtiness of genital secretions.

Young children have little opportunity to get hold of sexual facts or piece together the fragments they happen to acquire. Neither are they likely to link their fragments of knowledge to the only sexual fact they know enough to be curious about: the question of where babies come from. Children often have their own theories but hesitate to mention them simply because they can tell from adults' behaviour that it is best not to enquire too deeply. As one girl explained:

> Ever since I was about four I always wondered how you had a baby and so on — I had this weird idea that you just went to a doctor and he waved a magic wand and you had a baby. I suppose it did occur to me to ask — but I didn't have the nerve to do it.

Sometimes children keep quiet because they think their theories are right and do not need to be confirmed. It is accepted wisdom, for example, that when small children are told that babies grow inside their mothers they do not think about how they got there in the first place. I can remember my mother contradicting my grandmother's statement that babies fell from Heaven when I told her, being a sensitive five-year-old, that I was worried they might hurt themselves. I was quite satisfied with my mother's limited account because I already knew for certain how babies must come to be inside women. My grandmother could not have been entirely wrong; God put them there. A year or so later I heard some neighbours talking in hushed voices about an unmarried mother. I wondered how often God made such mistakes and felt that He ought to be more careful. My theory seemed quite satisfactory to me until my mother told me the whole truth when I was ten, not because I had come to doubt my vision of a careless God, but because I wanted to understand the jokes other children were telling.

If children do tell adults their theories they will often have them confirmed because people are unwilling to tell them the truth. This was one girl's experience:

> I always thought — well my mum told me you just took a tablet and you had a sort of balloon inside you and it just grew like that. I thought that and I asked her if that was right and she said it was.

Direct questions often do not yield any better answers. They may be met by evasiveness or a blunt refusal to answer, leaving the puzzled child wondering why so many things in the world are unmentionable.

The lack of sexual information available to children is itself a significant factor in learning. Already sex is being set aside as a special area of life — a secret preserve until the child is considered mature enough to know about it, usually at the onset of adolescence. This alone tends to give sex an air of furtiveness, and all the protosexual learning of childhood — the guilt, anxiety and 'dirtiness' associated with particular activities or parts of the body — can only serve to intensify the problem of coming to terms with new sexual knowledge.

When children stand on the threshold of their initiation into adult sexuality, most of their prior experience of it has been in the form of judgements and restrictions of their own behaviour. All they have learnt seems carefully contrived to make their subsequent sexual development as difficult as possible.

Girls and boys have been reared in different ways — to want different things from relationships, to gain pleasure from different sensations, to express emotions in different ways and to regard each other with suspicion and contempt. Since they will develop their sexuality through their sense of gender, their paths will continue to diverge, and yet they are supposed to bridge this gulf between them in their future sexual relationships, finding sexual pleasure in each other and so ridding themselves of all the guilt and anxiety they have learnt.

In expecting this of young people are we not asking the impossible?

7

Initiates and Novices:
Adolescent Sexuality

Adolescence is the most crucial phase of sexual development for most people in our society. The process begins with learning the basic facts of human sexuality, but much more than this must happen before young people can take on competent, adult sexuality. They must assimilate and make sense of the facts in terms of their own desires, emotions, behaviour and relationships. They must begin to cast themselves and others in sexual roles and learn how to establish and manage sexual relationships.

All this must be accomplished in a relatively short space of time: most young people will have been denied the opportunity to learn much of help in childhood so that, rather than gradually coming to terms with sexuality throughout their lives, adolescents find it suddenly thrust upon them. They enter this period of life still to a large extent sexually ignorant, and are expected to emerge from it sexually mature. This is one example of the strangeness of adolescence, an institution that few other cultures share. The existence of this transitional phase between childhood and adulthood creates confusion about exactly which childish or adult attributes young people should possess. With sexuality the problem is pronounced, since marriage, still the only fully legitimate form of sexual liaison, cannot be entered into until long after sexual and reproductive maturity has been reached. Although adolescents are recognized as capable of and interested in sex, the possibility that they might realize their potential or act on their desires causes adults many misgivings.

To complicate matters further, adolescence has no accepted boundaries; its beginning and end are neither fixed nor clearly defined. The beginning coincides more or less with puberty and is often assumed to be a consequence of it. But it is not puberty itself that propels the child into adolescence, for adolescence, even more than childhood, is a social institution rather than a natural psychological state. It is the acknowledgement of the effects of puberty that matters: the development of adult physical characteristics makes it difficult to carry on defining a young person as a child, and forces us to reassess her or him. The significance of physical events, such as hormonal changes, lies in the meaning they are given, for they are interpreted as signals that a young person is now capable of sexual relationships, and so should be treated in a different way. As with the onset of adolescence itself, individual sexual development does not seem to be affected by the rate of physical development as much as by social experience. There are many pre-pubescent thirteen-year-olds with well-developed sexual interests and many sixteen-year-olds, well past puberty, who are far less mature in this respect.

To become fully sexual requires knowledge of basic sexual acts. Again this knowledge is usually made available to young people at around the age of puberty, though rarely at exactly that time. Most people in Western societies discover the 'facts of life' between the ages of eight and thirteen, more often at around ten or eleven. Again the precise age has little to do with the individual's rate of physical development. When I talked to girls about their attitudes to sexuality I found no connection between the age when they first found out about sex and the age when they reached puberty, except in the few cases where parents prepared their daughters for the onset of menstruation and combined this with information about reproduction. However, the time when children or young people find out about sex may influence how they react. One of the few girls I talked to who remembered no negative feelings about sex said:

I can't remember a time when I didn't know. As soon as we asked questions we were told. I just learnt gradually — it was all very nice.

Significantly this thirteen-year-old displayed far fewer anxieties about sex than many older girls. Others who had learnt gradually also seemed to have accepted sexual knowledge without difficulty. But if information about sex comes as a sudden revelation, age is irrelevant. By far the most common reaction to first learning about sex among the girls I talked to was one of shock, often accompanied by disgust or revulsion. The following remarks were typical:

I thought it was 'orrible — but you've got to know, 'aven't you?

I was disgusted — I don't know why, I wasn't afterwards — it was just a shock.

I thought it was disgusting when I first found out.

I was shocked at first.

I thought it was dirty.

I thought it was horrid.

A bit shocked, yeah I think I was mainly shocked but, you know, you become accustomed to it and just accept it.

Shock is only to be expected when children are told about an aspect of life that has previously been carefully hidden from them. Although girls, being more thoroughly trained in the virtues of modesty and cleanliness than boys, are most likely to recoil from this new knowledge, the very suddenness of initiation probably means that boys will be shocked too.

Even if this new knowledge is imparted to children as a response to their own questions, their shock is not likely to be any the less. The one event of sexual relevance that cannot be concealed from children is the arrival of babies, and it is upon this that their questions are usually based. They are not asking about *sex* at all, but about an event of more general interest, and may be totally unprepared for the answers they receive. All children who learn about sex in this way are like the little girl in the well-known joke: 'Where did I come from?' she asks. Her mother takes a deep breath and launches into the biological details. 'Oh,' says the child, 'I only wanted to know because Jane said she comes from Newcastle.'

Sexual information is all the more difficult to

accept because it tends to be focused on the link between sex and reproduction. So children first learn about sex not in the context of their own feelings and emotions, not as a source of pleasure or as an aspect of human relationships, but as a means to an end. It is not presented as relevant to children's present lives, but something that will happen in the future, usually after marriage. This was how one girl felt about it:

I was a bit confused. I couldn't quite fathom it. It seemed a bit, well, peculiar, a dreadful thing to do. It was always something talked about after marriage, there was never any doubt about that. You get married, then you have sex, then you have a baby and that was how it was done.

Sex presented purely as a means to an end may seem odd or distasteful — a kind of surgical procedure submitted to in order to produce a baby. This sometimes leads children to believe that people only do 'it' when they want a child. Adults telling children about sex often mistakenly assume that this is the best way to go about it, the least likely to upset them; or they may simply be responding to questions about where babies come from. Often, sensitive to the possibility of upsetting children, they take pains to emphasize that this behaviour is 'natural'. Obviously this is preferable to conveying the impression, as many do, that it is all rather nasty and sordid, but such reassurance does little to balance the overall impression created by the reproductive emphasis, especially if sex is defined as something only married adults do.

One girl who was shocked when she first realized where she 'came from' had experienced the sort of initiation into sexual knowledge that is usually considered entirely satisfactory. As she explained it:

> My mother told me everything I needed to know. She said 'If your friends laugh at school and everything, just ignore them because it's only natural.' It had been talked about at school and I never understood what they were talking about — and so she just confirmed everything and told me it was natural.

The girl's mother had obviously taken some trouble to try to forestall any negative impressions of sex that might be gained from schoolfriends, but:

> When I was told about it my mother said, well, she just told me it was in marriage and I never really thought about it as being out of marriage.

The message this girl was receiving was rather confused: sex is 'natural' therefore acceptable (though there may be something more since others may laugh at it), but it is something that is only natural under certain conditions: when married people do it in order to have a baby. And for all her concern, this mother could not prevent her daughter being shocked. It is a pity that the few parents who talk to their children about sex are so often trapped into presenting it in this way. This can in no sense be blamed on the individual parents. It is, after all, accepted wisdom in our society that this is what children want and need to know. Children who find out about sex from other sources also tend to learn about it in reproductive terms, since all the information circulating among the young derives ultimately from an adult world in which sexual knowledge is thought to begin and end with the sex—reproduction link.

But we do not need to place so much emphasis on reproduction, even if that is what children ask about. We can tell them that pregnancy is a *possible* outcome of sex without giving the impression that this is *why* people engage in it. They might then find it easier to accept the knowledge, and we may even be able to counter some of the ill effects of earlier non-learning. The one girl I spoke to who remembered learning about sex as a pleasurable aspect of close relationships had this to say about her initial reaction to it:

> I wondered what it was like. I didn't wonder about the results of it, having babies and that — I wondered what the actual experience was.

Although those with puritanical views might find this alarming, this girl was spared the horror and disgust felt by so many of her contemporaries. I doubt whether conveying a negative impression of sex or stating that it only occurs in marriage is the best way of deterring the young from sexual activity: it is certainly not very effective. Many young people who first learn about sex in an unfortunate way do later become more sexually active than adults would like, and even if they do not, they will not necessarily share their parents' moral attitudes.

If we avoid overemphasizing the reproductive aspects of sex we can perhaps also prevent another common difficulty young people have in assimilating knowledge of sex. Just as Frankie refused to believe the 'lies' about 'married people' because they implicated her father and uncle and aunt, many young people find it difficult to accept that their parents must have gone through this rather distasteful procedure in order to produce them. Since this is something that has always been concealed from them, they are likely to view an integral part of their parents' relationship as funny, unimaginable or disturbing. If instead they found out about sex as something concerned with pleasure and affection, it would give them time to absorb the fact of their parents' sexuality without having it thrust upon them, and they might also find some features of their parents' relationship more understandable.

In thinking about these problems, I have come to be grateful that I was spared them. By some fortunate chance I found out about sex from my mother not in response to questions about babies but by asking her to explain the jokes that were being told in school. She did tell me about reproduction, but she also let me know that it was not an inevitable consequence of sex nor the reason for engaging in it. Like many other parents she was anxious that I should think sex 'natural', but she explained it in terms of attraction and arousal; I was told that I would feel these things and that sexual relationships were something to look forward to. All this was quite a revelation, but a pleasant one. Suddenly all manner of things that had puzzled me or that I had misunderstood fell into place, and most of all sex made sense in terms of my own feelings and experience. This approach to telling children about sex may not overcome all their anxieties, but it certainly helps. If, moreover, parents are able to convey the impression that they themselves are sexual and that they are willing to accept their children's sexuality, they might lay the foundation for a far greater degree of communication about

111

sexual matters than is usual between parents and children.

Parents are not on the whole very good sources of sexual information. Research on both sides of the Atlantic indicates that at most a third of girls, and less than ten per cent of boys, first learn of 'the facts of life' from their parents. There are several reasons why parents are more likely to inform their daughters about sex than their sons. Possibly girls, having learnt that it is they who can bear and rear children, are more likely to ask about reproduction. Most parents also feel it more necessary to prepare girls for menstruation than to inform boys about their physical changes, and perhaps they find it easier to impart sexual information in this context — although a substantial minority do not even tell their daughters about menstruation. It is also likely that mothers, who have more opportunity to discuss sexual matters with their children and are more often turned to for help and advice, find it more difficult to talk about sex to their sons. The willingness of parents (almost invariably mothers) to inform their daughters about sex may derive from the desire to protect girls and warn them against the dangers of pregnancy and sexual exploitation. Fathers do not feel it so urgent to inform their sons since it is assumed that they will find out about sex for themselves and will not be in any way endangered by it.

Most parents, however, offer little or no sexual information either to daughters or sons, yet there seems to be a general consensus that they ought to. I suspect that most parents want or feel they ought to be the people responsible for beginning their children's sex education, so why do so many fail to act? Again the chief problem is the secrecy that surrounds sexuality: how do you begin to convey information you have previously deliberately with-held, especially if it is something you feel uneasy about? Few people in our society can talk about sex as freely as they discuss other subjects. Many parents simply procrastinate, trying to preserve their children's 'innocence', postponing the day when they will have to accept them as sexual people, reassuring themselves that 'She's still a child' or 'He's too young to be interested.' As a result they often find they have been forestalled — their child has found out somewhere else. Among the girls I talked to, those whose first knowledge of sex had come from their mothers had learnt earlier than others: most had been aware of the link between intercourse and conception by the age of nine and all by the time they were ten. If it is left any longer it will simply be too late.

It might be easier for parents if children were more openly inquisitive. Although some parents refuse even to answer questions, many would be relieved if their children took the initiative in opening up the area for discussion. But many young people do not seek sexual information from their parents. By the time they are aware that there is something to be curious about, they are all too often also aware of its for-bidden nature. They may feel too embarrassed to ask, or fear that their parents will be unforthcoming. Sometimes these anxieties abate after a time, when young people have come to terms with the basic facts and their parents realize that they have been spared the task of teaching them. Then there may be opportunities for discussing sex, but in some house-holds it will still be unmentionable.

Since parents, usually the only adults that children are close to, are such unreliable sources of informa-

113

tion, young people generally have to fall back on their own resources. Most derive their first sexual knowledge from friends of their own age. Even when they have already learnt something about sex from their parents, talking to friends seems to be the main way of finding out more and making sense of what they know. Some may turn to books for help, a few might find school sex education useful, but for most young people these sources make little real contribution to sexual learning.

So young people pool whatever facts they have uncovered, exchanging knowledge among themselves. The circulation of information is restricted by age grading in schools, which reduces the chances of much of it filtering down to younger children. The move to secondary school in England or junior high in the United States is often significant, for here most people seem to encounter sexual information for the first time, having moved into a social setting where it is more widely available. Some of this information does cross the barrier into schools for younger children but seems only to reach the upper age bands. Children themselves help to control the flow of sexual knowledge through their awareness of age differences and tendency to choose friends of a similar age.

It is estimated that at least ninety per cent of young people's sexual knowledge is obtained from friends. But this is hardly a reliable method of learning: as many myths as facts may be exchanged, and much that is gleaned from whispered secrets and dirty jokes is only half understood. It sometimes takes time to assimilate even the simplest facts, and often children will look for further confirmation of what they have learnt before they will believe it. The final discovery

114

of what it is all about may come quite suddenly when all the pieces fall into place and the significance of past events is revealed. This is what happened to Frankie after her encounter with the soldier:

> she recalled the silence in the hotel room; and all at once a fit in the front room, the silence, the nasty talk behind the garage — these separate recollections came together in the darkness of her mind, as shafting searchlights meet in the night sky upon an aeroplane, so that in a flash there came in her an understanding.

Learning about sex in this way does little to dispel the aura of furtiveness that surrounds it, yet on the positive side, it does not seem to present sex in any more unpalatable a form than does any other kind of sex education. There seems to be little connection between how children find out and how they react to the new knowledge. Among the girls I talked to, those who had learnt from their friends were no more 'shocked' or 'disgusted' than those who had learnt from their parents.

The anxiety often expressed about the extent of young people's reliance on each other for sexual information may be misplaced. Only among themselves do most teenagers explore the implications of what they have learnt and consider its personal consequences. In linking facts with experience through their conversations with friends, they begin to dismiss some of the negative associations of sex, and, as they learn to establish relationships with boyfriends and girlfriends, they become aware of sexual activity as a potentially enjoyable aspect of them.

However much concern we may express about the

means of telling children about sex and about what they do with the knowledge, once they are told we offer little assistance. In coming to terms with their own sexuality and learning to manage sexual relationships young people are very much alone. At first sight girls seem to receive more help than boys. Most studies suggest that while very few boys receive advice on sex from their parents, the majority of girls do. On closer examination, however, this 'advice' consists of little more than moral injunctions.

Only a few parents openly discuss sexual matters with their children in such a way as to encourage them to make their own moral judgements and work through their own feelings about sex. This is not, after all, what most parents are seeking to do: they are generally more interested in handing down their own moral viewpoint. The usual advice to daughters takes the form of vague warnings to 'Be good' or 'Be careful', without any explanation of the sexual implications of the message. Often the consequences of illicit sex will be stressed, with references to girls who have a 'bad name' or who have become pregnant. Not infrequently parents seem intent on conveying totally negative attitudes to sex. This girls's experience is a common one:

My mother thinks it's dirty. She used to drum it into me from a young age that it was dirty. She said it wasn't nice, you know, out of marriage — I was told never to let a boy touch me.

This may be the sum of communication between parents and daughters about sex. As one girl put it: 'All I got from them was only what not to do.'

The reasons why girls but not boys are given these

moral directives are fairly obvious. Given the double standard that is still very much a part of conventional morality, girls must learn to guard their 'reputations' against those who view the sexually experienced as unworthy of respect. Girls are also vulnerable to sexual coercion and exploitation and the consequences of unwanted pregnancy. The anxieties parents have about their daughters are often based as much on well-grounded fears as on a false puritanism, but at the same time they offer girls little help in finding solutions. Nor do parents try to counteract in their sons the masculine attitudes and behaviour that cause such difficulties for girls. They might even reinforce the double standard by encouraging their sons to respect 'nice' girls, thus tacitly confirming that the rest do not deserve it. The attitude that 'boys will be boys' extends to an amused tolerance of the sexual exploits of the adolescent male. It is not unusual for parents, especially fathers, to admire their sons' sexual adventurism in secret, while at the same time trying to protect their daughters from the attentions of other people's like-minded sons.

This is all the help and support most young people receive from their elders in trying to make sense of sex and sexuality. Yet they have to strive to cope with a confusing and contradictory sexual morality and endeavour to meet each other half way in sexual relationships. To do so they must first overcome any negative feelings about sexuality and then try to understand the sexual desires and interests of the opposite sex. This is not an easy task and it is rarely completed successfully.

So how do adolescent girls and boys become sexual, and what are the consequences for relationships between them?

In order to become fully sexual young people have to develop an awareness of their bodies as a source of sensual pleasure. The links that young adolescents are able to make between their knowledge of their own bodies and the sexual information they have acquired are vitally important. The physical development of puberty and attitudes to bodily functions learnt in childhood combine with the reproductive emphasis of sexual information to ensure that boys easily become acquainted with the sexual capacities of their genitals while girls remain ignorant of theirs.

As we have seen, both girls and boys tend to learn about sex as a means to a reproductive end, but both will later realize that it is supposed to be pleasurable and can therefore be an end in itself. But by learning about sex as a reproductive act young people have also learnt to equate it with intercourse. Sexual intercourse is the 'real thing'; to engage in it is to 'go all the way' or 'get to home base'. Any other form of sexual activity is seen simply as a step on the way to the final goal or as a poor substitute for it: after all, even adult sex manuals call non-coital sex 'foreplay'.

All this makes it easy for boys to reconcile what they have learnt with their own experience of their bodies. The facts at a boy's disposal tell him plainly that the penis is his main sexual organ, and his experience of frequent erections, noctural emissions and ejaculation all fit in with the facts. At puberty his penis forces itself upon his attention and he is likely to explore its sexual function through masturbation, so that he has direct experience of physical arousal and orgasm and therefore some idea of the sort of pleasure to be expected from sexual intercourse. These experiences are frequently discussed by boys in their early teens, and although they may feel guilty or anxious about them they do at least have the opportunity to become aware of the potential of their sexual organs. In this way they create a basis for developing a sense of their own physical sexuality.

For girls the situation is quite different. Unlike boys they have not become familiar with their genitals during childhood, and most grow into adolescence still without direct knowledge of them, in particular, being unaware that they have a clitoris. Learning that sex is intercourse tends to mislead them into assuming that the vagina, the only sexual organ they know, is the focus of sexual pleasure for women. When I first began to talk to adolescent girls I naively thought that this form of ignorance would not be as widespread as it was in my own generation, but I discovered that still only a small number of girls knew about the clitoris and its sexual function, even among the more sexually experienced girls in their late teens. Many did not even know that women could reach orgasm, having equated it with ejaculation. So the information available to young people not only centres on reproduction but also reflects masculine priorities in defining sex as intercourse, an activity that virtually guarantees physical satisfaction for the male, but is at best a highly inefficient way of achieving it for his partner.

For those very few girls who have masturbated to orgasm in childhood, sexual knowledge will help them to understand what this means. Even so, they may still expect full pleasure from intercourse alone, and may be puzzled and disappointed when they discover that it does not necessarily involve the sensations they have come to recognize as sexual. For the great majority of girls, however, sexual satisfaction remains a rather abstract concept; not having experienced it, they have no idea what it will feel like. Girls have no experience parallel to boys' discovery of ejaculation, and nothing happens to draw their attention to the clitoris in the way that boys' attention is drawn to their penis. Few girls explore their genitals and few masturbate: the taboos they have learnt in childhood seem to hold them back. Many are horrified at the very idea, saying 'I wouldn't touch myself down there!' Even girls who do not declare any moral or aesthetic objections rarely try it. They often do not know what to do — which may be one reason why most adult women who masturbate begin only after someone else has done it to them.

The physical changes of puberty are more likely to draw girls' attention towards reproduction than sex. A boy might take frequent erections and ejaculation to mean that he can now 'have sex'; a girl will probably take the onset of menstruation and the development of her breasts to mean that she can 'have babies'. Menstruation is highly unlikely to be associated with sexual pleasure and may only add to a girl's negative feelings about her genitals. Developing breasts may have more sexual importance, as least as a sign of physical attractiveness, though few girls seem to feel this other than through anxiety about being over or under endowed. Some realize that the changing shape of their bodies arouses male interest, but this only makes them conscious of being sexually attractive, not sexually active.

Boys develop an interest in physical sexuality rather earlier than girls. Initially it is self-centred, and usually it precedes any feelings of sexual attraction, at least towards girls. If boys are to build on this foundation and move towards socially acceptable heterosexuality they need to develop at least a

120

minimal commitment to relationships with girls. This is not particularly easy for them. Their earlier training and rebuttal of all that seems feminine makes them wary of love and romance and disdainful of the female sex in general. Physical tenderness and affection are alien: it is easier for them to see any sexual relationships in terms of the masculine attributes they have already learnt to value. Acquiring sexual partners poses less of a threat to a boy's self-image if he regards it as an exercise in competitiveness and dominance than if he looks upon it as surrendering to feminine emotionality. This creates its own problems; if sexual activity with girls is proof of masculine prowess, lack of success can lead to feelings of inadequacy, especially if, as is common in boys' and mens' discussions of their 'conquests', the competitive element is foremost. But most boys in their early teens find the risk preferable to selling out to the effeminacy of romance.

Boys, then, tend initially to think of sex not as something they do *with* girls, but *to* girls. Later, though, they discover that they must at least get to know the romantic conventions if they are going to succeed in their conquests. Their earlier reluctance to learn these conventions is one reason why it takes them longer than girls to establish relationships with the opposite sex. For some, relationships will never be more than playing at romance — manipulating girls and persuading them into sexual intimacy. Most boys, however, do develop genuine romantic attachments in their late teens, but even then they rarely overcome their earlier feelings and attitudes completely. Often they can only maintain affection for a particular girl by placing her on a pedestal, idealizing her as different from all others. A boy in love can be even more romantic than the average girl, but it does not prevent him from having other sexual interests. A distinction is made between 'nice girls', for falling in love with, and the rest, ripe for sexual exploitation. Some boys are so trapped in this paradox that they can never reconcile love and sex — indeed this is one of the most common sexual problems adult men experience.

If for boys the idea of love does not easily fit with images of sexually competent masculinity, for girls it is a major way of reconciling femininity and sexuality. Through the allure of romance girls quite quickly overcome any revulsion towards sex and come to view it as pleasurable and an essential element in certain types of relationship. Most of the girls I talked to saw sex as an inevitable product of love and thought a good 'sex life' one of the most important factors in a happy marriage.

While girls do appear to overcome negative attitudes to sex, this does not involve any modifications in their knowledge of it. And just as boys learn that sex is something they *do to* girls, girls learn that it is something that is *done to* them. I was struck by the way the girls I talked to always spoke of sexual activity as what boys did to them, rather than what they did themselves, and I remembered that in our teens I and my friends had done the same. The sexuality girls are accepting can be summed up very simply:

sex = intercourse = something men/boys do to women/girls

This is hardly a very attractive view of sex, implying as it does an element of coercion, and denying the female any active involvement.

Most girls develop an apparently positive view of sex while continuing to think of themselves as sexually

122

passive and defining their sexual needs as centred on the vagina, complementary to the needs of the male. So they are not moving towards an autonomous sexuality through understanding their own physical potential, but are adapting to a male-defined sexuality with only a vague notion of the pleasure it is supposed to produce. The 'positive' attitude to sex that emerges during a girl's adolescence is in effect a passive acceptance of a form of sexuality that does not operate in her interests.

How does this happen? In one sense girls seem to be victims of a confidence trick so successfully contrived that they do not realize they have been conned. So long as they remain ignorant of the mechanics of female sexuality they will not realize that there may be more pleasurable alternatives to intercourse, or that boys, in striving for intercourse as the only goal, are depriving them of sexual satisfaction. It is difficult to remedy your ignorance when you are unaware of it. If by some chance girls do realize what they have been missing they are usually very indignant about the injustice they feel they have suffered. I am not suggesting that all this is the result of a calculated male consipiracy. No doubt most boys are as ignorant about it as their girlfriends. When (or if) they discover the truth they may even feel affronted by the apparent deceitfulness — after all, they must find it hard to believe that girls could be so ignorant about their own bodies.

The aspects of girls' sexual adaptation that cannot be explained by simple ignorance are more complex. It is here that romantic love comes into play, operating at several levels to make girls accept a form of sexuality that not only requires them to be passive but also leads them to think of their sexuality as a commodity,

123

an item for trade. But the ideals of love themselves produce certain ambiguities, so that girls are usually unable to develop an unqualified appreciation of sex as enjoyable in its own right. In defining sex as an act of love, girls can go some way towards accepting both sexual passivity and this view of their own sexuality as an object. If they think of sex as something done to them, they need not see it as undesirable if it is interpreted as a demonstration of the other's love. If they talk of sex, as they often do, as something they 'give' to boys, an object somehow detached from themselves, this is acceptable so long as sex is 'given' as a token of love and 'received' in the same spirit. Girls' common claim that sexual activity must be accompanied by love is more than just a moral statement: it implies that only through love can sex be transformed into an enjoyable experience. This girl expressed the feelings of many:

> If you love someone then it's all right. But there's a couple of girls who just sleep around, well, obviously that's just out. It makes the whole thing cheap and nasty instead of being a way of expressing your love for someone.

Lack of love pushes sex back into the realms of the sordid and distasteful; if love elevates sex, its absence debases it.

This attitude makes sex acceptable in the right circumstances, but it also creates considerable problems for girls. In order to establish that the correct conditions for sexual activity have been met, girls have to interpret boys' intentions, and they are fully aware that male motives for sex are often far from romantic. When girls complain that boys 'only

124

want one thing' or are 'out for what they can get' they are not mindlessly mouthing clichés but talking of something very real in their sexual lives. Nor are they simply denying their own sexuality when they imply that they do not want what boys want. Teenage girls have more wisdom than they are usually given credit for. They are well aware of the dangers of sexual exploitation and they know what boys think:

> Boys just want to prove themselves — they go and talk to a friend, you know, what they done with a certain girl and that.

No girl wants to be the subject of boys' crude conversations.

Girls have to believe that there are exceptions — 'not all boys are like that' — otherwise their romanticism could not persist. The problem is not only that sex is viewed as a symbolic act of love, but that girls' sexual feelings and arousal are all dependent on love. After all, they have learnt about sex in the context of romance, and even if they are experiencing what a boy would call lust, they are likely to identify their feelings as love. Further anxieties result: girls often feel vulnerable, being aware that they might be 'carried away' by romantic impulses only to find that the boy shares neither their feelings nor their commitment to the relationship. Part of the reason why girls insist on love before sex is that they fear boys will not make an emotional investment in the relationship; if they are 'out for one thing' they might disappear afterwards, while the girl has made a deeper commitment and placed her 'reputation' at risk.

The fear of a 'bad reputation' is constant: a girl needs to be sure a boy loves her so that she will not be talked of as a sexual conquest; she secures immunity from that humiliation with her place in the 'nice girl' category.

Beyond all this, of course, lies the fear of unwanted pregnancy and girls' knowledge that they could be deserted by the father of their child. Girls feel that if a boy loves them he can be trusted to stand by them, perhaps even marry them, should they become pregnant. Indeed, many girls take the precaution of extracting a promise of marriage before they engage in sexual intercourse. Boys know that they may be able to evade the responsibilities of an unwanted pregnancy, girls that they never can — in the end it is they who will have to cope with the consequences.

This situation is not helped by the difficulty young people experience — particularly if they are below the age of consent — in obtaining reliable forms of contraception. Freer access to birth control might help ease girls' problems, but will not solve them. In the first place, most teenagers live with their parents, who may refuse to accept their daughters' sexuality and want them to stay pure, so that the girls have to worry about keeping contraceptive pills or devices safely concealed. But there is also a deeper problem — girls' own reluctance to seek advice about contraception. Recent research suggests that this reluctance is closely bound up with romantic ideals and moral attitudes to sex.

Many — possibly most — girls and young women do not take steps to protect themselves against pregnancy until they are engaging in regular sexual intercourse. To seek contraception before then, in anticipation of their relationship becoming sexual, involves a degree of premeditation totally at odds with girls' views on love and sex. If sex is the product

126

of love, calculated forward planning is unthinkable. Sex is something that happens to them when they are swept away by an irresistible romantic passion. They feel it would be morally and aesthetically wrong to take precautions before sexual intercourse has occurred. Even girls who have already had an unwanted pregnancy often refuse contraceptive advice if they do not have a steady boyfriend, fearing that it would make them seem promiscuous.

Many girls find it difficult to see themselves as sexually active, even more so to acknowledge it to others, which they have to do when they visit a doctor or attend a clinic. They may fear meeting people they know at a clinic, or simply find it impossible to talk to medical staff without embarrassment. Because they have learnt to be passive and to expect the male sex to take the initiative it will be hard for them to take control of this part of their sexuality. Many just go on hoping, and sometimes believing, that pregnancy will not happen to them.

Boys are less bothered about preventing conception, and tend to assume that girls will take precautions since it is more important for them. Frequently the matter is not even discussed because young people do not feel enough at ease with each other and with their own sexuality. So each partner continues to avoid the question or regards contraception as the other's responsibility. A male friend told me recently about a young women who commented, after sleeping with him several times, that he never used contraceptives. Being used to women who took care of such things, he had assumed that she must be protected. Yet until then neither had mentioned the subject. In a relationship between educated adults, this is perhaps surprising; among adolescents, it is all too common.

The problem of contraception, then, is not merely practical but is bound up with the different attitudes to sexuality girls and boys develop and with the double standard these imply.

Underlying the whole issue is a great deal of confusion and ambivalence about female and male sexual needs. Young people are growing up in a society that is beginning to challenge the notion that sex is a male prerogative and to recognize that women too are capable of sexual desire. Most young people would probably accept these more modern views, but they often continue to believe that even if women do want sex, male sexual drives are more urgent.

Most of the teenage girls I have talked to have strongly asserted their interest in sex and their right to physical pleasure, but this feeling was tempered by their awareness that the boys were the hunters and they were the prey. They felt they were entitled to want sex, but to want it too much was morally suspect. Girls who were too interested tended to be condemned:

> Most boys want sex. I dunno, most girls want it too — some girls are right old slags and they want it all the time.

> If she just has sex with them for her own pleasure, you know, you can't think much of her.

Once more these attitudes come back to love. It is all right to want sex when it is associated with love, but to want it for its own sake is totally unacceptable.

Boys share in these contradictory attitudes. While they often seem to think they are victims of un-controllable lust, and they know it usually takes

128

considerable persuasion or pressure before a girl consents to their advances, they like to believe all the same that girls enjoy sex. A boy's sense of sexual competence rests not only on how many girls he can seduce, but on the quality of his performance: if the girl feels no pleasure his image of himself is threatened. Every girl and woman knows this, for her training in femininity suggests how she can fake excitement and orgasm convincingly. Ironically, girls who too obviously enjoy sex — or who are too convincing in their pretence — risk their valued reputations. Most boys feel that girls who are too willing or too passionate are suspect, and they may disdain prey that accepts its capture too keenly.

The problems of assessing the sexual needs and desires of the opposite sex are intensified by our natural tendency to assume that 'they' are reacting in the same way that 'we' are, impelled by the same motives, interpreting their emotions or sensations in the same way. Often girls will mistake a boy's look of passion for a look of tenderness. Boys assume girls are moved by lust when they believe themselves to be swayed by love. As a result girls who are over-romantic are often branded as too highly sexed.

This duality in female and male sexuality means that girls and boys unite in condemning girls who are too sexually active. Girls need to protect themselves by making it plain that they are more moral than others. Whatever the values of a particular group, there will always be other girls with whom they can compare themselves favourably. They do not resist the labels boys fix on them for fear of losing their own reputation — defending the promiscuous means you are counted as one of them. Boys, on the other hand, need to prove their masculinity through sexual activity, but they have learnt to despise anyone who gives them the opportunity to do so. Thus they too have an interest in maintaining the distinction between 'easy' girls and those they single out as objects worthy of love and affection.

It is difficult indeed for girls and boys to meet in honest enjoyment of their own and each other's sexuality, giving and receiving tenderness and pleasure without anxiety. Moreover, they are given little opportunity to overcome the obstacles that divide them. Engaging in sexual activity furtively, without the privacy adults enjoy, can only make sex seem sordid: it hardly gives young people the chance to assess their feelings about sexuality. The only young people who have the space and privacy to develop relaxed and regular sexual relationships are the privileged few at college or university, where they are free of parental supervision and childhood restrictions but not yet expected to take on adult responsibilities. Every survey of sexual attitudes and practices since the Kinsey Report has noted that among highly educated people there are fewer puritanical attitudes and double standards and a greater enjoyment of sex on the part of women than in any other sector of the population. This state of affairs is usually attributed to the effects of education, but I suspect it has more to do with the opportunities these people have had to come to terms with sex.

However, even giving young people more privacy and greater sexual freedom cannot do away with the problems they face. Most of my female contemporaries at university were overjoyed at the opportunities for sexual experimentation that this new environment provided. But we soon discovered that though we had plenty of time and space for sexual encounters, were

130

no longer damned for being sexually active and were freed by the campus clinic from the fear of pregnancy, all the other problems remained. The predatory male was even more in evidence, we still became emotionally involved while our partners did not, we found ourselves open to new pressures in the guise of the 'free love' ethic of the late sixties, we were hurt even more often, and we still didn't have orgasms! My male contemporaries probably have other tales to tell — of clinging, demanding women who expected too much of them, who deceived them by faking orgasms and later, rebelling, accused them of sexual incompetence.

Young people's problems in managing sexual relationships, problems that may well stay with them throughout adulthood and later be passed on to their own children, begin in the earliest days of their lives. The childhood training in sex roles, the conflicting ideas and feelings of adolescence, cannot easily be overcome. Greater sexual feeedom and easier access to contraceptives may alleviate some of their anxieties and difficulties but will not necessarily improve their lot, especially for girls. More freedom may simply make girls open to more sexual exploitation while the double standard persists, and there is no guarantee they will achieve physical satisfaction while sex itself continues to reflect masculine desires and priorities.

The sexual experiences young people undergo do not reflect merely gender differences, but a gender hierarchy; they are the product of a male-dominated society with a long heritage of patriarchal institutions, traditions, culture and values. Whatever problems boys may confront in coming to terms with sexuality, girls encounter more and suffer more in consequence. Whatever anxieties it provokes, male sexuality at least

131

gives the individual a sense of defining and controlling his own wants and needs. Female sexuality, conversely, is dependent on and defined by that of the male. Girls and women will not be able to develop a sense of sexual autonomy unless they cease to define their sexuality in reference to a particular loved man. Until then women will experience their sexuality not as their own but as something to be bestowed upon a particular man. This comment from a seventeen-year-old girl, talking about masturbation, seems to say it all: 'I wouldn't touch myself down there: that's for the man I marry.' An extreme case, perhaps, but one that sums up the problems our sexually divided society creates for young people emerging into adulthood.

8

Sex Education: Remedial Action?

How can we help young people as they struggle to make sense of sexuality and develop their own sexual relationships? One possible answer — and the most obvious one — is through some form of sex education. But this is a controversial issue, much debated but rarely agreed upon. Here, again, attitudes to children, sexuality and gender differences that are usually submerged rise to the surface.

No matter what our moral beliefs are, we tend to look on sex education as something of a problem. How much should young people know about sex? How do they find out? And what do they do with their knowledge? There is a wide range of views about the quantity of sexual information that should be available and the methods of disseminating it. Controversy is centred on a few main issues: does sex education increase or decrease the problems associated with adolescent sexual activity? Is it the responsibility of parents or schools? At what age should children receive it? Should it be confined to biology or should it include moral guidance too?

The effect of sex education on young people's sexual behaviour is often discussed as if it were something that could easily be measured. Both puritans and libertarians claim to have a monopoly on the truth, though they often reach their different conclusions by arguing from the same basic facts. One side declares that sex education has led to 'increased promiscuity'; the other denies it. Even if it were possible to pinpoint changes in teenage sexual activity, it would be difficult to establish to what extent sex education might be responsible. 'Increased promiscuity' could result from a variety of factors, including a broader change in society's moral climate. Sex education could merely be a symptom of this change, or it could have contributed to it. If sex education is said to encourage sexual activity, does this mean it portrays sex so attractively that it makes young people want to try it? This is absurd, but so is the counter-claim that sex education acts as a deterrent. Teenage pregnancy is another related issue. To some people the number of unwanted pregnancies is evidence of the ill effects of sex education, to others an indication that more is needed. Since sex education usually explains the link between sex and conception, if nothing else, it is difficult to see how it could promote teenage pregnancy unless girls actually want to become pregnant, which seems doubtful. But this does not mean that more advice on contraception would necessarily solve the problem; while young people are denied easy access to effective forms of birth control or are reluctant to use it there are still obstacles to be overcome. Further, as we saw in the last chapter, the failure to take adequate precautions against pregnancy seems to have more to do with young people's attitudes to and anxieties about sexual involvement than with sheer lack of knowledge about contraception.

When we anguish over who should provide sex education and at what age children should receive it we forget that this is a problem of our own making. If we did not hide sex from children in the first place neither of these questions would need to be raised. So arguments pass back and forth without our even mentioning, much less challenging, the strategies we use to conceal sex from children. That the choice of educators is so narrow is, of course, a consequence of children's isolation from the rest of the adult community, which then delegates responsibility to parents and teachers.

Whichever alternative is preferred, still more questions need to be raised. If sex education is fixed within the sphere of parental duties, what happens to those children who receive no sexual information from their parents — the vast majority? Should they be left to their own devices? If this drawback leads, as it often does, to the conclusion that school sex education is the only workable alternative, how do we fit it into the curriculum? Sex is not easily slotted into the usual categories of teaching. In these debates the third possibility — learning about sex from friends — is rarely considered, for it is generally dismissed out of hand as inadequate. This response is so ingrained that the reasons behind it are seldom explained. Yet most people find that even if they are often misinformed, their friends provide more useful and relevant information than either parents or teachers.

The 'facts' versus 'morals' debate is largely irrelevant. Sex education can *never* be divorced from moral values. Even if sex is reduced to its biological facts, the selection and presentation of those facts implies moral messages. For example, a description of the sexual organs could emphasize either the reproductive or the sensual functions, thus conveying quite different images of sex. Moreover, all debates on sex education revolve around its supposed effects on the young, revealing that we are not simply seeking to offer them information but are interested in influencing their behaviour.

It is hardly surprising, given the confused state of public debate, that formal, school-based sex education has, in most Western countries, developed in a rather haphazard fashion without any clear rationale. It has been seen as a regrettable necessity, created out of the uncomfortable knowledge that sexuality is very much a part of adolescents' lives and the fear that they may not acquire the right sort of information in any other way. There is wide agreement that the family is the appropriate place for sexual learning, but since so many parents abdicate responsibility educational authorities see it as incumbent on themselves to remedy the deficiency. Most young people seem to agree. Among the girls I talked to, few learnt anything from school sex education but they were unanimous in considering it a good idea, if only for the benefit of those who had not learnt about sex elsewhere.

While both teachers and students agree that some kind of formal sex education is desirable in the circumstances, only the former have any say in deciding the content, timing and method of teaching. Except in countries with comprehensive national programmes, such as Sweden, there is no clear policy, so that sex education varies greatly from one school to another. In the United States over half of all public and parochial schools have sex education programmes and federal funds are available for developing them further, but there is still considerable confusion about

136

their purpose. They are justified as encouraging healthy sexual attitudes without much explanation of what this is supposed to mean, or as preventing teenage pregnancy without much thought as to how to achieve this. In Britain, funding for sex education is hard to come by, and while most schools might claim to offer some sexual information to their pupils, only a small minority have anything like a continuous, comprehensive programme. While government reports have recognized the need for sex education for decades, and local education authorities issue guidelines for schools, neither say precisely what its purpose should be or how its content should be defined. Usually such official documents refer vaguely to the need to educate young people for marriage and parenthood and encourage responsible attitudes to sex; there are often moralistic statements too, such as this one (quoted by A. Harris in 'Sex Education in Schools') from the Inner London Education Authority's guidelines:

Sexual intercourse should never be seen as a transient pleasure but as a joyful consummation of close friendship, love and understanding which in marriage have time to grow and deepen.

It is clear from this and the many similar statements that British educators see sex education as preparing adolescents for the future rather than helping them to come to terms with sexuality here and now. Its chief aim, indeed, is apparently to dissuade them from expressing their sexuality at all. The dangers of sexual activity are consistently overemphasized: while most schools tell their pupils about venereal disease, only a minority deal with contraception; most head teachers believe it should have no place in sex education. It looks as though young people are told about the risk of disease not to help them recognize the symptoms and seek treatment, but to deter them from sex. As in the United States, sex education is often justified as a means of preventing illegitimacy, but given the usual lack of advice on birth control it appears that the main strategy is the preaching of abstinence accompanied by dire warnings about the diseases that afflict the unchaste.

The United States seem to be moving away from this morbid preoccupation with the unfortunate aspects of sex. Whereas in the sixties educators were accused of dwelling on the perils rather than the pleasures of sex, they are now being attacked for their mechanical and impersonal approach. If this is true the criticism is deserved — but at least American teenagers have the chance to learn about the ways of deriving physical pleasure from their bodies. In the majority of British schools this is still unthinkable.

The British approach to sex education offers young people little of immediate relevance; for girls the avoidance of the issue of contraception may be disastrous. Some of the more comprehensive programmes currently followed in the United States may be more helpful, even if they do concentrate on physical responses at the expense of emotion. But there are some encouraging trends in recent literature on both sides of the Atlantic: it is now emphasizing the need to relate sex education to young people's experience. It remains to be seen whether this is effective; despite some teachers' keenness to put such ideas into effect, the restrictions imposed by educational institutions make the task a difficult one.

Teaching sex education in schools does have the

advantage that it has the potential to reach all young people — a captive audience. Yet it is precisely because of this that problems arise. The school, an institution children are forced to be part of, where adult control over them is at its most overt, is not the easiest environment for encouraging free discussion of sexual matters. Pupils are likely to be fully aware that their attitudes and behaviour may be disapproved of, and too conscious of teachers' authority to talk openly. Moreover, the adolescents whose sexuality causes most concern tend to be those classed as 'deprived' or 'difficult'. They are often thoroughly disillusioned with an education system that offers them few rewards, and are hardly likely to be receptive to teachers' advice on how to run their lives.

Teachers, on the other hand, are acutely aware of their responsibility and that they too are vulnerable to authority, and may as a result feel uncomfortable about discussing sex in their classes. Sexual experiences are considered deeply private, and are rarely discussed freely and honestly except with intimate friends, if at all. This is problem enough in itself, without the further complication of worrying about young people's sexual behaviour — fearing that it is all too easy to encourage them to 'go too far'. So to start up discussions on sex within the authoritarian climate of the school is no easy matter. Though sexuality is a personal matter, it is precisely here that personal experiences are least likely to be aired. Teachers may illustrate a French or geography class with anecdotes about their holidays in France, say, but if they talked about their sexual encounters in France to illustrate cultural differences in behaviour it would be considered shocking.

Teachers who do take a personal approach to sex

education may find themselves in trouble. Not long ago a young teacher in England became the centre of a public scandal for just this reason. In an attempt to encourage a class of sixteen-year-olds to examine the double standard of morality and male sexual exploitation, he wrote a description of how he felt about girls and sex when he was their age. He used the language that he and his friends had used at the time, and that the pupils were likely to use themselves. This enterprising attempt to break down the barriers between teachers and taught and discuss a vital aspect of adolescent sexuality was damned by higher authorities as obscene and corrupting. In daring to talk about subjects that were actually relevant to young people's sex lives he forfeited his job, and it is unlikely that any school will employ him now.

Most teachers are not prepared to take this kind of risk. Understandably, they play safe, and so ensure that sex education remains detached from their own and their students' experience. Even if they were not held back by the fear of losing their jobs, many would find it difficult to do otherwise. Education in general is organized around 'academic' knowledge, something quite separate from everyday life. Even when the topic is close to personal experience — talking about the family in a social studies class, for instance — pupils are encouraged to 'transcend' their subjective outlook and adopt a new, objective perspective. So despite the fact that the whole rationale for sex education is that sex is or will be part of students' lives, links between facts and experience are rarely made. If they were, teachers would have to abandon the usual conventions of academic knowledge, accept their pupils' choices for discussion, and be prepared to work through rather than against personal experience. Even if a teacher accepts this, it is not likely that he or she will easily develop the kind of relationship necessary for such open discussions with pupils when it is discouraged in other subjects.

Taking a personal approach also undermines the teacher's status as a purveyor of knowledge — in the realm of personal relationships he or she will have no more expertise than any other adult. In sticking to the 'facts', and planning sex education lessons as they would any other class, teachers avoid this threat. New answers to this particular problem — to make sex education a subject in itself, or to invite outside 'experts' into schools — will probably make matters worse. The most popular outside speakers are traditionally doctors: granted, they may know more about the physiology of sex than most of us, but they are no more informed about sexuality as a whole, about managing emotions and relationships, than anybody else. Now there are attempts to extend this expertise further, in training teachers and doctors as specialists in human sexuality.

At first sight this looks like a liberal move: often such training focuses more attention on sexual pleasure and relationships, topics usually excluded from more traditional teaching. But this school of sex education, now becoming popular in the United States although still not accepted in Britain, rests on the justification that it promotes 'sexual health', thus extending the claims of medicine beyond its rightful boundaries. The effect is often to make sexual relationships seem more of a minefield than adolescents already know them to be, superimposing a new set of anxieties on existing ones. It is absurd to suggest that anyone can tell us how we ought to have sex. Young people are hardly helped to talk about their sexuality if they fear they may be judged unhealthy as well as immoral. In schools, this teaching seems to imply that there is a right way to 'do' sex as there is a right way to do algebra, sex having correct solutions just as simultaneous equations do.

So what are the effects of placing sex education in the hands of the experts? Not only is sex again divorced from experience, but an assumption arises that we need experts to tell us how to have the right sort of experience. But how can anyone be an expert on human sexuality? People who have read widely or thought a lot about the subject may have ideas that can be shared with others, but that does not necessarily make them any better at handling their own sexual relationships, and it is sheer arrogance to presume to dictate to others. Sadly, though, it is unlikely 'experts' will merely share ideas in schools — they are liable to try and impose their beliefs on those they teach.

The trend towards making sex education a specialist field of its own may partly be a response to the difficulties of integrating it into the normal school curriculum. Education as we know it largely consists of presenting pupils with packages of knowledge in the form of the various subjects, each separate from the rest and each presented as a body of objective facts. Turning sex education into a subject in itself and disguising moral issues as medical is one way of placing it on a par with physics or history. But is it right that young people should regard sex as being just as detached from their daily lives as other school subjects?

Before this new development there were two main possibilities, both still practised today: teaching sex education within an established school subject, such as biology or religious education, or setting it aside as a special event outside the usual school routine. Neither is very satisfactory.

The first option means that the scope of sex education will be limited by the boundaries of the subject within which it is taught. If it is brought under biology, the most frequent choice, it will be reduced to the anatomy and physiology of sex differences, conception and birth. If relegated to the relative backwaters of physical or religious education, or social studies, it will be presented in terms of health, morality or family structure. Nowhere is it likely to be directly related to pupils' experience. There is no reason, though, why sex should not be discussed within the usual school subjects: after all, it may crop up not only in the subjects I have just mentioned but also in such fields as art, literature and history. Indeed, it might help to break down the barriers between sex and the rest of life and encourage young people to discuss it less self-consciously if this did happen. If biologists looked at the physical processes, teachers of religion discussed the moral and ethical issues, historians covered changing attitudes to sex, social scientists considered contemporary patterns of attitudes and behaviour, art and literature teachers looked at portrayals of the erotic, all this might help young people appreciate sexuality as simply one aspect of life. Perhaps the discussions would still not be directly related to pupils' own feeling and experiences, but they could be interesting and informative, dispelling the notion that sex is something special and apart.

In practice, however, sex is 'done' within only one or two subjects, and only by teachers who have been given special responsibility for it. Sex is usually deliberately excluded from the rest of the curriculum, and any relevant material — say in history or literature — is reserved for pupils nearing the end of their school career. Here again teachers might find themselves in trouble if they infringe the unspoken rule. A history teacher I know was reprimanded by her headmistress for informing a class of thirteen- and fourteen-year-olds that Edward II was homosexual. Her defence, a just one I think, was that it was impossible to understand the political conflicts of his reign without this knowledge. What she ought to have done, apparently, was allude to 'close friendship' rather than admit his homosexuality. How absurd that such censorship should still take place — that while we conceal sex from children in some lessons we should then have to worry about how best to reveal it in others.

The 'special event' tactic may avoid the limits of teaching sex education within only one school subject, but has difficulties of its own. The very fact that it is taught outside the normal curriculum points up the slightly risque nature of the enterprise. There will probably be speculation, joking and giggling among the pupils about the forthcoming entertainment, the school having implied that it is unusual and clandestine. The effect is heightened by the ritual of sending letters to parents requesting their permission, the result of school authorities' anxiety about presenting sex to pupils where it cannot be justified as an essential part of an academic subject.

The same fear of causing offence will guarantee that the occasion fails to live up to pupils' expectations; the information they receive will be limited and probably tell them little they do not already know. Decisions on the content of sex education often make allowance for the most conservative moral viewpoints.

Frequently all that is offered is an outline of reproductive biology, perhaps accompanied by a moral lecture on the virtues of marriage and the risk of disease for people who indulge their lusts outside it. My own experience of school sex education was very similar. When I was sixteen we were shown a film which, with the aid of brightly coloured diagrams, informed us of the mechanics of conception. Afterwards the girls were given a talk on the virtues of chastity and the boys were told about contraception and venereal disease. We girls clearly did not need to know about this. There are still many schools which offer nothing better.

Problems like these might be avoided by making sex education a subject in itself taught to children throughout their lives. At least it would be possible to discuss many aspects of sexuality, and perhaps the aura of 'specialness' might be dispersed. In Sweden programmes along these lines have been run in all schools since the 1950s. A handbook for teachers issued by the Board of Education says:

> At no stage should sex education appear as something sensational or remarkable. Therefore it should be incorporated as part of a continuous course in which it has a natural place, without being given a special position.

For this reason mixed classes are the rule. It is felt that, while some children and young people might feel less inhibited in single sex groups, this would ultimately cause more difficulties by making lessons on sex different from other classes.

Although the Swedish system has distinct advantages, it would prove difficult to implement in

Britain and the United States. Sweden has a small population and few ethnic and cultural divisions. In Britain and the United States, on the other hand, schools are dealing with children who come from a wide variety of racial, cultural and religious backgrounds, so that the chances of offending some part of the community are greatly increased. This is not a problem to be dismissed, nor one that is easily resolved. It might seem unjust to put children so much at the mercy of their parents' beliefs that they are denied an education that could be useful to them. We do not cease to teach geography because members of the Flat Earth Society object to their children being taught that the world is round, yet here, as with sex education, we may place young people in the difficult position of having their parents' beliefs challenged at school. Perhaps children themselves should be offered the choice, but it is not always easy for them to decide whether they want something they have never experienced. For most people sex *is* something special, something they feel they ought to be consulted about when it concerns their children's education. A national system of sex education imposed by the state on communities that do not want it smacks of totalitarianism, especially as sex is so closely bound up with ethical and political concerns. Do we want an official sexual policy foisted upon our children?

In many schools in the United States, comprehensive sex education programmes have been put into effect without parents having been consulted or given the option of withdrawing their children, and this has sometimes caused great public protest. In many schools, though, the fear of provoking such a response has ensured that the scope of sex education is less ambitious. In Britain, where school authorities are rather more cautious and where education has always been a key political issue, most schools stick to traditional styles of sex education.

The result of British caution is an extremely erratic pattern of sex education. A few schools teach the basic facts of conception before children reach puberty, but for the most part it is not until after they have gone on to secondary schools that they are taught anything about sex. Here responsibility is often delegated to individual teachers or left to the discretion of teachers as a whole. The outside speakers who most commonly appear are doctors and officials from the Public Health Department; more adventurous schools invite speakers from birth control clinics. Usually sex education consists of one lesson or one or two talks or films. In talking to girls who attended five different schools I discovered a distinct lack of planned, coherent courses. Two schools put on programmes for third formers (thirteen- and fourteen-year-olds) but they were confined to one year rather than being part of a continuous process of learning. In one other school first form pupils were shown a film about conception and birth (described by one girl as consisting of 'a matchstick man here and a matchstick woman there') as the sum total of their sex education, except for the few pupils who had lessons with a particular woman teacher who encouraged discussions on sexuality. In the other two schools there was no sex education at all other than in examination biology courses, which dealt with reproduction.

It is hardly surprising that schools contribute so little so sexual learning. If the aim of education authorities is to replace other young people as the main source of sex education they will have to offer much more than they have so far. Schools may not be able to provide the opportunity for linking facts with experience in the way young people can among themselves, but perhaps they could supply information that is difficult to obtain elsewhere or encourage discussions between boys and girls on matters that are usually only talked about in single sex groups. As it is, though, sex education adds little to what young people already know about sex and rarely helps heal the breach between the sexes; it may even make matters worse because of the way it is usually defined and its implicit or explicit sexist bias.

Sex education is frequently reduced to little more than an outline of reproductive biology, implying that what adolescents need to know are the facts of conception and reproduction, a view rarely challenged. Yet most of this information is not really vital. Obviously young people ought to know that sexual intercourse is likely to lead to pregnancy unless adequate precautions are taken, but the finer details are generally superfluous to their immediate needs. We hardly need precise knowledge of the digestive system in order to organize our diet effectively, so why is it thought so important to understand fertilization, implantation and foetal development before we can manage our sexuality? Obviously the way our bodies work has its own fascination, and the development of a new human being may be particularly interesting, but most of this knowledge is quite unrelated to adolescents' day-to-day experience of sexuality.

Within the framework of reproduction, sex is presented as part of a larger sequence of biological, rather than social, events. More emphasis is placed upon biological processes than on the subjective experiences of sexual activity. The typical imagery is summed up by sociologists John Gagnon and William Simon in *Sexual Conduct* as that of 'the noble sperm heroically swimming upstream to fulfil its destiny by meeting and fertilizing the egg'. Not only is this unrelated to the feelings and experiences of adolescents; it also portrays the female function as entirely passive. The egg can never be heroic: it just waits around for Supersperm to arrive. Women's bodies are mere receptacles for the man's penis and the growing baby. The language we use to describe intercourse makes the same point: we speak of 'penetration' of the woman's body, or the 'insertion' of the penis into the vagina.

As long as sex education is so defined its content will mean little to young people except in so far as it confirms the stereotypes of male activity and female passivity. As it is conventionally taught it has little to do with *sexuality* but is confined purely to *sex* — biological 'facts' rather than emotions and relationships. When it is confined to reproductive sex it becomes even more divorced from experience.

Some of the material used in sex education lessons makes this clear. One handbook for teachers, Julia Dawkin's *A Textbook of Sex Education* (now, thankfully, out of print, although it is still to be found among the meagre stock of sex education books available in teacher training establishments), includes the following information in a lesson for ten- to twelve-year-olds:

> The penis, as you know, is for getting rid of liquid waste, but it has another use when a man is married: it is used for fertilizing eggs.

149

Quite what this is supposed to mean to an adolescent boy on the verge of discovering orgasm and ejaculation the author declines to say; it is as if the penis lies dormant, springing to life only after marriage, when it is called upon to dispense sperm. She does, however, hint that there might be something more to it:

Sexual intercourse is a very special way in which husbands and wives show their love for one another.

But sex is depicted as an entirely mechanical operation, and the description of fertilization that follows shows that this is its real purpose.

Another consequence of a reproductive bias is that it does nothing to remedy girls' ignorance of their own sexual response. The only female organs worthy of consideration are those involved in reproduction, so that the clitoris is rarely mentioned and normally is not shown on diagrams of 'sexual organs' (actually reproductive organs). The textbook quoted above informs girls that they should know the correct term for the ovaries, uterus and vagina, but fails to mention the external genitalia at all and ignores the role of the clitoris, even in the sections on classes for older children. There the author follows the usual line on masturbation, saying that it 'should always be discussed with boys' in order to avoid guilt over a natural process. However, since 'it is far less common in girls it need not be discussed'. But girls are entitled to know (though only if they ask) that it will do them no harm.

This is a common pattern. Male masturbation is worth mentioning because it can be described in biological terms, female masturbation is not. Male orgasm is usually covered as it is necessary for conception, female orgasm is not. Thus female sexual organs and orgasms are seen as irrelevant. Boys are at least told that the penis is their main sexual organ; girls are misinformed, told that the vagina is theirs. The assumption is that sex is important to girls only as it affects their future role as wives and mothers. So they remain ignorant of the means of deriving pleasure from their own bodies, given information only on their reproductive, not their erotic, potential.

The trend in recent years has been to provide sex education for both sexes, to begin it earlier, and to go beyond reproductive biology. Even so the starting point is still reproduction, as in Sweden, for example, where more ambitious courses are the rule rather than the exception. Books provided for younger age groups almost always have titles like *Where Did I Come From?* or *A New Baby*. Sexual pleasures may be mentioned and cute pictures included of smiling mummies and daddies engaged in sexual romps, but the message is still the same: the real purpose of sex is reproduction.

Of course, in purely biological terms, this is true, but the meaning of sex goes far beyond this. The justification for taking reproduction as a starting point is that small children find it fascinating. So they do, and they are entitled to have their curiosity satisfied. But this is not education about sex but merely about the functions of the human body, and children are fascinated about other aspects too — for example, what happens to food after they have eaten it. Young children could equally be taught about sexual pleasure, and not just as if it were something only adults enjoy — that would be downright dishonest. Why not teach them all about their bodies? The body's senses are interesting to young children;

151

why not include the sensuality of the genitals too? Once more, discussion of sexuality in all relevant contexts could be the best way of helping children accept it as just one more aspect of life.

One reason why sexual pleasure has so often been excluded from sex education is that educators have long been fighting a rearguard action against those who fear that modern youth is being corrupted by over-exposure to sex. Reproductive biology at least has the advantage of not being erotic. But whether teachers tell them or not, young people find out for themselves that sex is supposed to be pleasurable. The reproductive bias of what they have learnt at school is highly misleading for girls. Believing that intercourse is the peak of sexual activity, they might be tempted to taste its forbidden fruits when more accurate information could suggest other possibilities. Perhaps nature, having endowed women with separate sexual and reproductive organs, has provided them with a means of birth control. If one reason for sex education is to prevent unwanted pregnancy, would it not be helpful to tell girls about the sensual potential of their bodies, and let both boys and girls know that it is possible to give and receive sexual pleasure without engaging in the act of intercourse?

Such are the values of our culture that non-coital sex is often thought 'more obscene' than sexual intercourse: in some states in the US, for example, the law still defines oral sex as a perversion. Moreover, people charged with the care and education of the young seem to have deep fears of the consequences of discussing sexual pleasure as anything other than a side effect of reproduction. At one point I talked to many girls at a youth club and initially had the full knowledge and approval of the staff, who all spoke about the deplorable state of sexual ignorance among the young. They were aware that many of the girls who came to the club were sexually active, and were keen to offer them as much information and advice on contraception as possible. But when they discovered that I was talking to the girls about such subjects as sexual arousal and orgasm their reaction was almost hysterical. The youth leader called me into his office and delivered a tirade about the evils of encouraging the girls to be promiscuous. He could apparently accept that the girls were engaging in sexual activity and should be protected from un-wanted pregnancies, but found the prospect of their enjoying the experience appalling.

People who worry that information on sexual responses might be so arousing that it leads to instant promiscuity seem to have little cause for alarm if American sex education programmes are anything to go by. Most of the description of arousal and orgasm uses highly clinical and detached terms. Like the more traditional form of sex education it is remote from feelings and experience. Some people have attacked this mechanistic approach, arguing that it reduces human beings to sex machines whose reponses can be triggered by pressing the right buttons. The tendency to present sex education as a pre-packaged set of facts (one difficult to overcome in schools) and to imply that healthy sexuality can be objectively defined, may mean that these new approaches to the subject make future generations slaves to a stress on performance. On the other hand, programmes like these include vital information not readily available elsewhere, information to which young people need to have access.

We should, however, avoid presuming to tell them how to use this knowledge, or implying that only certain forms of sex are 'healthy'. To do so again avoids the emotional dimension of human sexuality, concentrating too much attention on organs and orgasms. It strengthens the goal-oriented attitude to sex: the idea that each time should be the perfect earth-shattering experience, anything else meaning failure, so that sex is once more a focus for anxiety. If we exchange the notion that sex is dirty and sordid for the notion that it must be ecstatic every time, we do not seem to be making much progress.

I have been arguing that information on the female sexual response is necessary to redress the bias of young people's sexual knowledge, but knowledge itself is not enough to change the nature of relationships between the sexes. It will take much more than this to make the average male rethink his ideas about sex. One of the things that struck me most forcibly about the *Hite Report* was that the women who discuss their experience in it seemed exceptionally knowledgeable about and well adapted to their own sexuality, and yet were still, for the most part, unable to make use of their awareness in heterosexual relationships. Men were still imposing on them their idea of the right pattern of sexual activity, culminating in intercourse. If adolescent girls knew how their responses work, it could help them enjoy sex more but does nothing to solve the most pressing problems facing them, the double standard and sexual exploitation by men. If boys are being taught that arousing girls is simply a matter of stimulating the right organ, it might even make them more callous about exploiting girls' vulnerability.

The only way to confront this problem is through

discussion of girls' and boys' feelings about each others' sexuality. Many young people who cannot easily start up such discussions themselves might find this useful. Perhaps it could also help overcome one of the major inadequacies of sex education, presenting sex as a mechanical exercise remote from individual experience. Among the girls I talked to, the most common criticism of their sex education (other than that it told them nothing they did not already know) was that it excluded emotions and relationships.

Unfortunately, when sex education does go beyond facts to explore the meaning of sex and feelings about it, sexist bias tends to come to the fore again. Instead of examining critically the double standard of morality and the stereotyped ideas about female and male sexuality that underpin it, sex education tends to reinforce them. I suspect that it is here that teachers are most likely to turn for guidance to books by 'experts', feeling that their own experience is inadequate. Certainly the sale of sex education books cannot be accounted for simply by the very small number of young people who read them. Most of these books, whether for adolescents or teachers, tend to over-emphasize the differences between the sexes and make all manner of assumptions and generalizations about them. One such expert, a Dr Eleanor Schill, stresses the need for boys to understand female sexuality in the following terms:

> It is not always easy for a man . . . to understand her (often unconscious) desire for pregnancy as a result of intercourse when for him the relief of tension is the more important aspect.

In the same book, ironically called *Honesty to*

Children, the editor, F.G. Lernhoff, argues that sex education should begin before puberty, saying:

> it is especially important for boys to know the further implications of the woman's role in sex and how it is linked with homemaking and motherhood and her whole emotional life before their own sex-drive becomes too persistent.

This book is not a voice from the distant past, but from the early seventies. The contributors do seem to be looking backwards, though, for they recommend as the best book available for young people K. Barnes's *He and She*, written in the 1950s and hopelessly out of touch with young people's lives today though still, unfortunately, widely used in Britain. It offers such gems as:

> until she is married and deeply roused by all that marriage means, the desire for sexual intercourse is not very strong in a girl.

More recent books often offer similar ideas. P. Perry's *Your Guide to the Opposite Sex*, published in 1970, tells boys that:

> You should not for a moment think that girls have no physical sexual sensations at all.

Well, this is some kind of progress. But he goes on to say:

> These sensations are different from yours in that they tend to be rather vaguely spread throughout the body and seem to most girls just general

156

yearning feelings — rather like looking at a beautiful sunset and wanting to keep it but not knowing how.

This is supposed to be a description of physical arousal, not romantic love. If young people are being presented with this sort of nonsense it is no wonder that boys feel girls who enjoy sex too much are somehow morally suspect, and that girls, protective of their reputations, condemn their more sexually enthusiastic sisters.

Even books that are otherwise quite informative tend to advance rather dubious ideas about female sexuality. W.B. Pomeroy's *Boys and Sex* and *Girls and Sex*, popular in both Britain and the United States, are better than most. Yet *Girls and Sex* offers its readers the following piece of advice:

> It may take a girl weeks, months or even years after marriage to unlearn what she has been taught about being 'a lady' . . . . for a full and happy married life, she must learn to respond in the bedroom while she maintains a ladylike appearance the rest of the time . . . It is important for girls to understand this dual nature of their lives as soon as possible.

Pomeroy has here hit on an important source of conflict, one I have already identified as causing problems for girls in coming to terms with their sexuality. Advising girls to be whores in the bedroom and ladies elsewhere, though, is hardly much help. This issue could have been the basis for a critical exploration of sex roles and sexuality, asking, for example, why sex should seem unfeminine, a useful

157

discussion point. Pomeroy, who seems to suggest that this female sexual schizophrenia is somehow inevitable, avoids the issue.

Fortunately, a few much better books are beginning to find their way onto the market. The best I have come across is Jane Cousins' *Make it Happy*, which despite its rather coy title is honest, straightforward and tackles most of the specific problems of sex education that I have discussed. Jane Cousins always sets sexuality in the context of emotions and relationships, discusses many ways of giving and receiving sexual pleasure without suggesting that there is one correct method, and combats many false assumptions about the nature of female and male sexuality. She offers clear and accurate information on almost everything young people might want or need to know about. If anything, the book is organized rather too much around problems, but as adolescents do face so many difficulties this is perhaps unavoidable.

The approach adopted in *Make it Happy*, which is now beginning to be used in schools, also counters another bias written into most sex education programmes: they have traditionally been not only sexist but also heterosexist. An outcome of the overemphasis on reproduction and sex-as-intercourse is that non-heterosexual relationships will be defined as unnatural. Homosexuality is rarely discussed; where it is, it is often labelled a perversion or treated as a passing phase in sexual development. This perspective does not help those who are attracted to others of the same sex, nor will it make young people any more tolerant of homosexuals and lesbians. If sex is portrayed as a pleasurable way of relating to others, rather than as a means to a reproductive end, homosexuality might be seen as just as valid as heterosexuality. Indeed, it might be worth considering the claim made by many homosexuals and even more lesbians that their relationships, devoid of the elements of power and exploitation that characterize heterosexuality, are *more* valid.

Most educators, though, would probably want to avoid this, for they are even more wary of encouraging homosexuality than 'promiscuity'. Even the new forms of sex education that emphasize sexual response still tend to define homosexuality negatively. Bound up with medical models of sexuality as they are, these new approaches simply provide a new reason to disapprove of homosexuals and lesbians: they are 'sick', not perverted. Perhaps this promotes greater sympathy, but sympathy and tolerance are no substitute for genuine social acceptance.

It is this tendency to make sexuality a medical matter that seems to be undermining the advances made in the United States. Ideals of sexual health and stress on the technicalities of performance again set sex aside as a special area of life — the focus of a new set of anxieties. Realizing this, sex educators are going round in circles, and now begin their courses with therapeutic sessions intended to encourage an easy interchange of ideas. So we have books like E.S. Morrison and M.U. Price's *Values in Sexuality*, intended for use with college students, which begins with a section on 'group building activities' that is full of statements about discovering 'anxiety and discomfort provoked by a course on sexuality' and 'reducing selfconsciousness and inhibition'. They tackle this problem by asking students to sit on tables in groups of six and discuss how they feel about touching each other. Will this really reduce selfconsciousness? Certainly, to begin a sex education course in this way does little to challenge the idea that there is something unique about the whole enterprise. Have we really, as this book implies, arrived at a state of affairs where young people need remedial psychotherapy before they can hope to attain a 'mature sexuality'?

I suspect that this remedial approach creates more selfconsciousness than it cures and encourages people to see problems where none exist. This trend towards therapeutic sex education is now being extended to adults. First in the United States, and more recently in Britain, people who are prepared to believe that they have any problem experts may diagnose have become entitled to pay enormous fees for the privilege of being subjected to 'cures'. One such course for men in Britain offers participants the opportunity of spending a day watching films on masturbation, after which they split into pairs and describe their penises to each other. Whether they feel this helps them I could not say. But do we really need these experts telling us whether or not we are sexually 'healthy', and making huge profits from what they define as our problems? Are we really so damaged that we need therapy?

The sexual therapy movement is a logical outcome of a long tradition of remedial-style sex education. We should recognize that schools can never provide a full education in human sexuality; we are expecting too much of teachers if we ask them to take on a responsibility that the rest of the community has avoided, to solve a problem that the whole of society has created. None of the difficulties surrounding sex education would exist if we did not treat children as a special category of people and sexuality as a special area of life. The best that schools — a product of the

160

former practice — can do is to try to challenge the latter. The way to do this is not through formal, separate sex education programmes, but through discussing sexual matters wherever they are relevant, in all areas of the curriculum and throughout children's school careers. The problem, once again, is not how to tell children about sex, but how to stop concealing it from them.

9

Women and Children First:
Protection or Oppression?

In raising questions about sex education I have returned to one of the central themes of this book: the way in which sex is concealed from children. The fact that formal sex education exists and that it is the centre of so much controversy is symptomatic of a major problem concerning children and sex: that after consistently hiding an important aspect of social life from young people, we then have to face the difficulties of lifting our censorship.

I have argued that the attitudes underlying contemporary anxieties about children and sex are confused, ambiguous and founded on many false assumptions. In particular, as I showed in chapter 2, much of the debate concerns the influence of 'nature', assuming that childhood is a 'natural' state and sexuality a 'natural' form of behaviour. Ideas about naturalness have confused our understanding of the typical patterns of sexual development in our society. One side in the moral debate talks about the dangers of repressing children's sexuality, the other of the need to preserve their natural innocence. Libertarians complain that the strategies we use to keep children sexually ignorant are 'bad' for them; puritans lay

162

claim to their beneficial effects. Both, however, base their arguments on 'nature'. I would agree with the libertarians that the present state of affairs is harmful, but not because it violates the true nature of the child. Instead I have based my evaluation on the difficulties children and young people encounter as a result of the concealment of sex from them, on the way this emphasizes the low status of children and their segregation from adult society, and on the undesirability of depicting sex negatively and subordinating women. The problem as I see it is not the *repression* of basic drives but the *oppression* of women and children.

In arguing against 'naturalness' I have criticized the way in which sex is treated as a special area of life and children as a special category of people. Obviously this is not because I think they are unimportant — if I did I would not have bothered to write this book. Sexuality *is* an important area of social life. It is closely related to the most fundamental of social divisions, that of gender, and to one of the most basic social institutions, the family. Childhood is an important stage of life precisely because so little of human behaviour is natural; it is in our early years that we learn what is expected of people in our society. What I am concerned with are the consequences of our beliefs about the special nature of childhood and sexuality.

One of these consequences, highly significant in itself, is that children learn so little about sex before they reach puberty. In concealing sex from them we seem to be suggesting that it is dangerous or unpleasant. Indeed, we live in a society with a long tradition of moral opposition to sexuality, where sexual desire itself has often been regarded as immoral: after all, lust is one of the seven deadly sins. Within certain forms of Christianity — a major influence in shaping our culture — even sex within marriage has been regarded as morally suspect, and a recent Papal declaration has reaffirmed its sinfulness. This explains why innocence is equated with sexual ignorance. If the key to sexual knowledge is seen as the link between sex and conception, is this not because reproduction has traditionally been the only 'pure' motive for sex? These attitudes have been by no means completely eroded. Despite all the recent talk of the need to promote healthy sexuality, children are still being reared in a moral climate that is hostile to sex.

They are also being reared in a society divided by gender, in which anti-sex attitudes have been closely associated with misogyny. For instance, many sexual terms are used as insults and expletives, the most common being those for the female sex organs. In medieval times, the idea that women were responsible for men's degradation through lust was made explicit. Today a similar viewpoint is still to be seen in the way boys and men feel it necessary to denounce and degrade women who too easily allow them to satisfy their sexual desires. Since sex is so often a cause of guilt, it is not surprising that men should try to displace their feelings on women, and because we live in a society where men have shaped the laws, morals and values, they have usually succeeded in doing to. This guilt, emerging as hostility towards women, finds its expression in sexual exploitation and coercion, threatening not only women but also children.

Children in our society grow up wary of the opposite sex. Long before this mutual suspicion is incorporated into sexual relationships, they learn to conform to ideals of femininity and masculinity that would make it difficult enough for them to like and trust each other even if power, male dominance and female subordination did not enter the picture. Girls and boys develop opposed values, attitudes, emotions and behaviour, and yet are expected to unite as adults to establish a lasting bond in marriage, an institution based very firmly on sexuality. The consequences are neatly summed up by the English feminist Lee Comer:

> Any glance around society reveals that the sexes are placed on opposite poles, with an enormous chasm of oppression, degradation and misunderstanding generated to keep them apart. Out of this, marriage plucks one woman and one man, ties them together with 'love' and asserts that they shall live in harmony and that they shall, for the rest of their lives, bridge that chasm with a mixture of betrayal, sex, affection, deceit and illusion.

It is in childhood that we begin to travel along the paths that lead to this gulf between men and women. There we begin to mistrust each other and to learn to be the dominated or dominant partner in sexual relationships.

Clear parallels can be drawn between the status of women and children, and also between the stereotyped images of them that our society generates. Just as children and adults tend to be portrayed as polar opposites, so do women and men. It is not only that what is feminine or masculine, childish or adult is summarized through opposites, but that the two sets of stereotypes overlap. What is adult is frequently equated with what is masculine, and what is child-like with what is feminine. So both women and

165

children are supposed to be passive, dependent, vulnerable and emotional; adults and men, meanwhile, are active, independent, aggressive, competitive and logical.

An apt example of this tendency is provided by a study of American clinicians' ideas as to what constitutes mental health. Psychiatrists, clinical psychologists and psychiatric social workers were given lists of characteristics and asked to indicate which they thought typical of 'normal healthy adults', 'normal healthy men' and 'normal healthy women'. There was widespread agreement: the depiction of the healthy adult proved identical to that of the healthy man, while the attributes considered typical of the healthy woman were virtually the opposite. It seemed that in order to be considered normal and healthy, women had to be dependent, emotional, vulnerable and childlike creatures.

If the normal, adult human being is by definition male, then the female of the species, given our tendency to think in opposites, is not quite normal, not quite adult and not quite human. Ideas about maturity are thus associated with gender, so that there is a contradiction between what maturity requires in itself and what female maturity demands. While boys are expected to shake off the shackles of dependent childhood, girls are expected to retain them, progressing from a girl-child to a child-woman. As well as the usual economic reliance of women on men, they are expected to develop a psychological dependence which they share with the very image of dependence, the child. Just as children are thought to need adult protection, so are women in so far as adult equals male.

This may well explain the commonplace observation

that girls mature earlier than boys. They have less to mature into — maturity for them being little more than a superficial gloss on their existing childish attributes. Hence the English upper-class myth of the finishing school, wherein the gawky schoolgirl is transformed almost overnight into a sophisticated young lady by virtue of a few lessons in dress and deportment. Consider Agatha Christie's description of the murder victim in *Sparkling Cyanide*:

> Schoolgirl Rosemary; clumsy, all arms and legs. 'Finished' Rosemary coming back from Paris with a strange new . . . elegance, soft voiced, graceful, with a swaying, undulating figure . . .

The much vaunted 'mystery' of femininity is largely this: a veneer of sophistication over a basic childishness.

The history of the ideal of vulnerable feminity runs parallel to that of the vulnerable child. In the middle ages there was no doubt that women and children were social inferiors; both lived under the strict patriarchal authority of men. Yet neither were considered fragile incompetents, and both were expected to work for their living, even among the upper classes. Wives of the aristocracy and gentry were quite capable of managing the estates while their husbands sought power and glory in innumerable wars and crusades. For the lower orders life was hard irrespective of age and sex and long continued to be so. Men showed little inclination to protect women and children from hardship and, indeed, had few means of doing so. The up-and-coming bourgeois man of the seventeenth century still wanted a competent wife to help him run the business, and trained his children early to pull their weight. His successful nineteenth-century counterpart wanted his wife to be an 'angel in the house' to soothe his troubled brow, a decorative ornament shielded from the grim realities of life to serve as a visible symbol of his success. He also wanted wide-eyed, innocent and cosseted children to complete the picture. While his daughters were educated in schools that advertised the fact that they took pains not to overtax the delicate constitution of the fair sex, the women and children of lower classes were still working in gruelling conditions in mines and factories. When the first protective legislation was introduced to limit working-class child labour it was accompanied by similar provisions for women, and gradually 'protectiveness' began to filter through the class system until 'women and children first' became a slogan accepted by all. Working-class men soon wanted angels and cosseted children in their houses, too, as symbols of rising living standards and respectability. The trend was to exclude both children and women from the real world — to confine both within the family so that woman's childlike nature was emphasized by her physical proximity to her children and her interests were identified with theirs. The exclusion of children from adult (especially male) society and the creation of special institutions for them was paralleled by the growing conviction that 'a woman's place is in the home', an idea that is actually fairly recent, though it is often associated with the past.

Until Victorian times small boys were dressed like girls and wore their hair long. When their curls were cut and they were dressed in masculine clothes, their progression from the feminine status of child to the masculine status of adult was made visible and obvious. This practice also served to express clearly what was (and still is) expected of boys in their passage to manhood: the abandoning of all things feminine and childish. Small boys are not necessarily eager to do this but are placed under considerable pressure to conform. They soon learn that they must at all costs avoid being cissy or babyish. This is to be branded as failures, too much like the inferior caste of females to be fit company for their brothers. In order to avoid this ostracism and maintain their self-esteem they have to steel themselves for battle in the harsh, competitive, aggressive world of the adult male. If, as sometimes happened, a Victorian boy cried when his curls were shorn, he would be sternly told that such behaviour was unseemly, for now he must 'be a man'. Today the transition is less abrupt, but the message is the same.

Among the childish attributes that boys must sooner or later grow out of is that of asexuality. Since childhood and femininity are so closely connected it is not surprising that both have become de-sexed. As part of our anti-sex heritage woman have always had a dual image as virgin and whore, but the emphasis has shifted through history. The chief reason why women were more vulnerable than men to accusations of witchcraft was that, in the words of the witch hunters' manual, the *Malleus Malefecarum*: 'All witchcraft comes from carnal lust which in women is insatiable.' But in the long journey from the lusty wench of the middle ages to the asexual Victorian 'lady', the virgin never quite supplanted the whore, just as the innocent child never quite exorcized the demonaic child. The two-sided image of women has usually been resolved by dividing women into the good and the bad, with ideal femininity being equated with asexuality. In the nineteenth century, the morals of the factory girls were suspect because they were 'unladylike', that is, more independent than was thought desirable. Even today the mature feminine woman is supposed to be barely sexual, at least in public. Now, though, each woman is supposed to resolve the contradiction within herself, with 'experts' like Pomeroy recommending whoredom in the bedroom and ladylike behaviour elsewhere.

For boys the emergence of active sexuality is one sign of their growing maturity, evidence of the break with the asexual passivity of childhood. Signs that a girl is growing up are usually taken as her interest in — and ability to attract — the opposite sex. But, as I have already pointed out, the mature young woman is supposed to be sexually *attractive*, not *active*. Part of the allure of femininity depends on sexual desirability matched by unattainability. A woman must appear attractive but unavailable until such time as a man wins possession of her, when she must become constantly available to him but not to anyone else. The asexual Victorian lady could be imprisoned for denying her husband his 'conjugal rights'; the modern woman is still supposed to remain pure but be eager to satisfy her husband's demands. So, while children are not supposed to be sexual at all, women are not supposed to be autonomously sexual but to express their sexuality only in response to the needs of a particular man.

It is through keeping children asexual that we prepare the ground for the emergence of the passive, dependent style of sexuality expected of adult women. If we did not keep children sexually unaware and prevent them becoming sexual, it is difficult to see how half of them could be dissuaded from sexual activity and independence as they grow into adults. It

170

is far easier to keep all children asexual and then encourage boys towards active sexuality (as we do) than it would be to ease the process of becoming sexual in childhood and then persuade girls that they must surrender it. Feminine and masculine sexuality reflect the wider demands made of femininity and masculinity in our society. Just as maturity for men depends on a relinquishing of childishness, so their sexual maturity means abandoning childlike asexual innocence. Not so for women. Their transition to adult sexuality requires little change of them beyond agreeing to sexual acts, and this is worked by their attraction to romance and their desire to please others, characteristics that are developed early in a girl's life.

For boys the achievement of sexual maturity requires a much sharper break with childhood. The passage to active, adult male sexuality is not always a smooth one. Boys must strive for (or be driven towards) a form of sexuality where they are always the active partners in sexual encounters. It is they who have to take the initiative, make things happen and control the event; it is they who must 'perform'. The penalty of being the doer rather than the done-to is the everpresent possibility of failure. As a boy grows towards manhood he learns that sexual conquest is an important but risky means of proving his masculinity: he must cope with the fear that he might not meet the accepted standards and be judged as 'less than a man'. The sexual arena is also — like many other spheres of male endeavour — a highly competitive one. The knowledge that his sexual performance will be measured against that of others only serves to intensify a boy's anxieties, and these feelings may stay with him throughout his adult life.

The modern performance ethic demands not only that men should perform often but that they should perform well. A successful man should be able to satisfy as well as seduce. At the same time he must appear to be in control; any display of emotion, of such childlike or feminine qualities as dependence, tenderness or gentleness, may indicate that his partner is controlling him. For many boys and men the need to prove themselves through sex while maintaining a semblance of emotional distance from their partners can be a constant source of anxiety and confusion. It is this that leads them to seek partners who are more emotionally vulnerable and less sexually experienced than themselves, who pose no threat to their fragile sense of sexual competence.

It is not surprising, then, that feminine attractiveness is so closely identified with childlike qualities, that vulnerability and dependence, coyness and cuteness all enhance a woman's sexual appeal. One reason why ideals of female beauty emphasize youth so strongly is that only young women can exploit these childish attributes to the full. It is usually considered rather grotesque for a forty-year-old to 'play cute'. The appeal of childlike qualities is most evident in men's tendency to be attracted to women much younger than themselves, even by immature girls, a tendency that finds its most extreme expression in the schoolgirl fetish so frequently exploited by pornographic materials. Not many women are attracted to men much younger than themselves; fewer still are turned on by pubescent boys. Schoolboys are certainly not erotic, and I find it hard to imagine any woman being aroused by pictures of men dressed up as schoolboys complete with short pants and school caps! It is easy to see why men find childlike vulner-

172

ability so appealing: having learnt to be sexually aggressive and dominant, they find it easier to play out this role with a partner who is passive, submissive and relatively powerless.

The facts that men learn to associate sex with power and develop the capacity to be aroused by childlike qualities creates the possibility that their sexual interests could be directed towards children themselves. Child molesters and child rapists are almost invariably men who have learnt to express their sexuality through aggression, to seek power over others and to be attracted to the vulnerable. The man who molests little children, if he is not brutal and sadistic, is not particularly 'sick' in comparison with 'normal' men. His desires and motives are probably much the same as those of the office boss who seduces his secretary, the lecturer who goes to bed with a succession of young students, and all men involved in similar relationships where male power is reinforced by institutional hierarchies.

But this association between sex and power makes violent sexual assault a constant possibility, and the victims are almost always women and children. It is because sexual coercion is such a prominent feature of relationships between men and women that children, too, are placed at risk. In a society where sexual relationships are not expressed through activity and passivity, aggression and submission, dominance and subordination, sexual assaults on both women and children would be inconceivable. The only reason why women and children need protection from sex is because men have learnt the arts of sexual coercion and exploitation so well.

Adult rape victims are often seen as responsible for their fate, though children's innocence usually goes unquestioned, for the sexual demon within is not usually thought to have played a part. The 'innocent' adult victim — the one that the police are likely to believe, the one whose aggressor the courts are likely to convict — is she who conforms best to asexual, child-like standards of femininity, she who is clearly dependent on a father or a husband, the virginal daughter or the faithful wife. Children are by defini-tion childlike and therefore always innocent victims. Yet maybe they do not seem so to their attackers; perhaps these men do perceive the sexual demon within. Nabokov's hero in *Lolita*:

> had the utmost respect for ordinary children, with their purity and vulnerability, and under no cir-cumstance would he have interfered with the innocence of a child . . . But how his heart beat when among the innocent throng, he espied a demon child.

All this man is doing it extending to girls the double standards generally applied to adult women. For the 'guilty' adult victims of sexual assault are those who do not conform to childlike femininity, who dare to be sexually active and behave as though they were self-governed. In eschewing the protection of a particular man they have declared themselves the property of all men and abandoned their claim to protection by the patriarchal institution of the law.

Children are protected by the law because they are always under adult (male) protection and control. Here again children's asexuality and women's lack of sexual autonomy run parallel. If children are kept asexual, this not only makes it possible to keep women sexually passive, but also symbolizes children's subordinate status, likens them to women and defines them as part of the feminine world. Even before women were regarded as asexual, chastity was still regarded as the ultimate feminine virtue: men's control of women's sexuality has a long history. Women's sexuality was protected by men because they sought to control it as they would any of their property. Medieval law makes this explicit; rape was seen not as a crime against a woman but as the theft of male property, and the law required that compensation be paid to the wronged husband or father whose property had thereby lost its value. That is why today only a woman whose value has not been diminished by sexual contacts is considered worth protecting. Women still use their sexuality to bargain for economic, social and emotional security, and know that to do so they must remain relatively asexual — the value of the commodity they are exchanging depends on it.

The relationship of women to their sexuality has been likened to that of a trustee to someone else's money. Lorenne Clark and Debra Lewis put it like this:

Prior to marriage, a woman's sexuality is a commodity to be held in trust for its rightful owner. Making 'free' use of one's sexuality is like making 'free' use of someone else's money. One can act autonomously only with things that belong to oneself. Things held in trust for others are surrounded with special duties which place the trustee under strict obligations for the care and maintenance of the assets in question . . . women are not regarded as being entitled to use their sexuality according to their own desires because their sexuality is not theirs for the use of such purposes. Their duty is to preserve it in the best possible condition for the use and disposition of its rightful owner.

Kept childlike, women do not become autonomously sexual but come to see their sexuality as something detached from them, a precious gift to be offered to a man prepared to pay the appropriate price. Boys learn to treat female sexuality as a commodity too, but they also learn that through sex they establish rights of ownership. Boys and men talk of 'possessing' a woman, 'taking' or 'having' her. The act of sex becomes a means of establishing rights in a woman as well as dominance over her.

As children, boys share in feminine asexuality. While they remain dependent and vulnerable they are not thought worthy or 'ready' for sexual autonomy, and are judged to need protection from adult male sexuality in the same way as women and girls. But as boys emerge from this feminine world and begin to progress towards manhood, their growing independence is matched by the development of their sexuality. They learn that they will now take on the role of sexual protector, controller and exploiter.

In absorbing this lesson boys too come to view their sexuality as detached from themselves, but this sense of detachment is very different from that experienced by girls. Girls may view their sexuality as a commodity but they nonetheless feel it to be inextricably tied to their deepest emotions. Success in the masculine role, on the other hand, requires a rationing of tender feelings. In shying away from romanticism and from the involvement of his whole personality in sexual experience, a boy will often

176

learn to distance himself emotionally from his sexual acts. In so doing he comes to focus his attention solely on intercourse and to think of his own sexuality as something concentrated in his genitals. His sexuality is thus externalized and projected onto his penis, which comes to be seen as an extension of himself, rather than as an integral part of himself.

This penis-centred sexuality simultaneously adds to and helps defend against the anxieties created by the demands of performance. In placing so much emphasis on the penis, boys become obsessed with its qualities, and may even continue to be anxious about its size as adults, fearful that they may be under-endowed and thus compared unfavourably with other men. They worry also about their ability to obtain or maintain erections, for proof of their masculinity rests on this above all. To be impotent is to be powerless — the two words are synonymous — and that means being unable to express dominance through sex. Yet in concentrating their sexuality in their genitals boys and men can distance themselves from the penis, think of it as a 'tool', and therefore protect themselves against possible failure. A man who can't get an erection would rather express his condition as a failure of his penis rather than a failure of himself, and many of the slang terms available enable him to do just that. To say that he 'can't get it up', for example, implies that 'it' — the penis, the tool — has failed him rather than that he has failed.

Viewing the penis in this way, men can distance themselves from any uncomfortable contacts with women. They can insulate themselves against the threat of being engulfed or contaminated. If they feel any guilt about sex itself, or any revulsion towards the female body, they can reassure themselves that only a small part of their person is implicated. At the same time they can feel that they have acquitted themselves well if the penis has done its job. Thus, despite all the anxiety about performance, few men are trying to please women but rather to convince themselves that their penis is as good as any other man's. Either they assume that what they regard as a good performance will be appreciated by the woman, or they do not even think about it. Men confronted with complaints from women about sex are often genuinely perplexed. 'But it was all right for me' is the usual response — meaning, of course, that it should automatically have been all right for you too. If the tool works properly, all should be well.

In thinking of the penis as a tool with which they do things *to* a woman men can further retreat from the consequences of a relationship. Thus they rush towards sexual intercourse rather than waste time on more sensuous pursuits of the kind that require greater rapport with their partners. It is often noted that while women prefer sex at night, men prefer it in the morning. Women have learned to enjoy the sensuous intimacy of falling asleep in a lover's arms, but for some men this is threatening. Better to wake from the relative anonymity of sleep, engage in a quick bout of sex and then escape from intimacy to the male-dominated outside world. As Phyllis Chesler said in *About Men*, summing up what men had told her about their sexuality:

Men, upon being questioned about their enjoyment of sex, almost seem to be saying that what they enjoy *most* about sex with women is having it over with, especially when they feel they've acquitted themselves well. Acquitted themselves of any doubts about their virility or ability to 'perform'. Acquitted themselves of the sin or itch of lust . . . Acquitted themselves of their need for a woman — for an inferior and dangerous being . . . Acquitted themselves of any charge of nonmasculinity . . .

This is just the sort of sexuality we seem to be educating boys for. The more masculine they are, the more successfully they are directed away from such 'feminine' or 'childlike' qualities as gentleness and tenderness, and the more they become emotionally stunted beings, unable easily to give and receive affection. Growing boys learn that sex is supposed to be enjoyable, but their need to dissociate it from feminine emotionality, to use it as a means of proving their masculinity, and to localize it in their genitals all limit the pleasure they could gain.

In learning this kind of sexuality men not only limit their own sexuality, but deny sexual autonomy to women and children, and so create the need to protect them. If men come to see the penis as a tool, it is only a short step to regarding it as a weapon. If using it effectively is associated with dominance and with proving their prowess as men, they may be tempted to employ it as an instrument of violence. The temptation will be greater the more a man avoids femininity, for he is then less likely to be able to empathize with women and children as fellow human beings.

The paradox that women need to be protected *by* men because they need to be protected *from* men has led feminists to realize that the rhetoric of male protectiveness is merely thinly veiled oppression, an aspect of male control and power. This has made women

179

aware of the need to redefine their own sexuality in ways that neither conform to nor mimic masculine priorities.

Given the connections between the status of women and children, the ideas of the women's liberation movement should help us to raise questions about the status of children and the adult power wielded over them, and to consider the possibility of redefining *their* sexuality. It is because we keep children dependent, vulnerable and asexual that women come to share these qualities. It is because only the male sex learns to break free from these bonds that men become more autonomous than women. It is because male autonomy is associated with power and aggression that men maintain control over women and that the need is created to 'protect' women and children. We need to question whether our apparent concern for children, our protectiveness towards them, is just a subtle form of oppression, as it is with women. It is these concerns that ought to guide us in assessing current attitudes to children and sex and their effects on the young.

I began this book by talking about breaking taboos. I will now commit the final heresy by stating clearly my belief that we do more harm than good in enforcing sexual ignorance on children. In attempting to protect children from sex we expose them to danger, in trying to preserve their innocence we expose them to guilt. In keeping both sexes asexual, and then training them to become sexual in different ways, we perpetuate sexual inequality, exploitation and oppression.

This is not merely a plea for greater sexual 'freedom' for children. Although in many respects I am drawn to this view, I cannot give it unqualified support. It is difficult to envisage sexual freedom within the present structure of society. As individuals, we may be able to create conditions in which the children under our care have less difficulty coming to terms with sexuality, rearing girls to be more independent and boys to be less aggressive, but these children still have to fit into society as it is, although they may ultimately help to change it. Only collectively can we overcome the problems of a society divided by gender and founded on competitive, acquisitive values that extend to sexuality. If sexuality, as I have argued, is not an isolated aspect of social life, we cannot expect it to change in isolation, nor can we expect to change anything merely by individual effort. Sexuality is not just a personal issue, but a political one.

We may not be able to change the world overnight, but we can begin by changing the attitudes of future generations. We can start by communicating more openly about sex and ceasing to conceal our own sexuality from young people. We must also avoid imposing our own preconceptions of femininity and masculinity upon them. We must stop encouraging boys to be tough and aggressive, and teach them to value gentleness, affection and tenderness instead. Then, perhaps, they would learn to appreciate a more sensuous, less exclusively genital, style of sexuality, and would not view their sexual organs as tools or weapons. They should also, in coming to value more highly the characteristics now thought of as exclusively feminine, be able to treat women and girls as fully autonomous human beings, not as objects to be possessed and dominated through sex. At the same time girls must not be prevented from gaining knowledge of their own bodies. They might then be able to explore their own sexual potential, rather than viewing their sexuality as a gift for a loved male. They must be encouraged towards independence rather than passivity, to seek their own goals in life rather than serving those of men. They would then be better equipped to resist having their sexuality defined by men, and could begin to think about defining it for themselves.

I cannot deny that this will be difficult. Parents and teachers who are trying to make changes can testify to the problems, not least the attitudes of people resistant to change. But if we do not try we are colluding in the perpetuation of sexual coercion and exploitation, of sexual guilt, of the oppression of women and children.

There are no easy solutions. Because we inhabit a society where sexuality is inextricably bound up with power and dominance, where the weak may be sexually exploited by the strong, where sexuality itself is exchanged as a commodity, true sexual freedom for children — and indeed for all of us — can only be illusory. It will remain a dream until sexuality is divested of its competitive and aggressive elements, separated from property and ownership, and no longer contributes to the subordination of women and children. And that, for the moment, is perhaps only another vision of utopia.

Further Reading

A full bibliography containing all the sources I have drawn on would run to several pages. Instead I list below a few books that others might find interesting and informative. The other works I have referred to in the text are listed in the References.

Philippe Ariès, *Centuries of Childhood* (Cape, 1962; republished as a Peregrine Book, 1979).
> The classic history of childhood.

Robert Brain, *Friends and Lovers* (Paladin, 1977).
> An anthropologist's view of sexual and other relationships, explicitly critical of contemporary Western attitudes to love and sex.

Phyllis Chesler, *About Men* (Women's Press, 1978).
> The Essay on Men that appears at the end of this book offers some interesting ideas on male sexuality and sexual development. My male friends assure me that it is far more revealing than anything written on the subject by men.

Jane Cousins, *Make it Happy* (Virago, 1978; republished by Penguin, 1980).
> The best sex education book currently available. It is aimed at teenagers but could also give parents some useful hints on how to talk to their children about sex. Unfortunately, there is nothing I could unreservedly recommend for younger children.

John Gagnon and William Simon, *Sexual Conduct* (Hutchinson, 1974).
> An approach to sexuality which differs radically from the psychoanalytic tradition, and one that has influenced me a great deal.

Shere Hite, *The Hite Report* (Dell Publishing Co., 1976).
> A detailed study of the way women feel about their sexuality. It says little about childhood experiences but should provoke some reflections on how both girls and boys learn about sex.

Martin Hoyles (ed.), *Changing Childhood* (Writers and Readers Publishing Cooperative, 1979).
> An interesting collection of articles and poems about and by children, and a useful starting point for anyone interested in childhood and children. The articles are well referenced for the benefit of those who would like to delve deeper into the subject.

References

R. Ardrey, *African Genesis* (Collins, 1961)

K. Barnes, *He and She* (Darwin Finlayson, 1958)

L. Clark and D. Lewis, *Rape: the Price of Coercive Sexuality* (Women's Press, Toronto, 1977)

L. Comer, *Wedlocked Women* (Feminist Books, 1974)

M. Douglas, *Purity and Danger* (Routledge & Kegan Paul, 1966)

J. Dawkins, *A Textbook of Sex Education* (Blackwell, 1967)

A. Harris, 'Sex Education in Schools' in R. S. Rogers (ed.) *Sex Education: Rationale and Reaction* (Cambridge University Press, 1974)

P. Laslett, *The World We Have Lost* (Methuen, 1971)

F. G. Lernhoff (ed.), *Honesty to Children* (Shotton Hall, 1971)

B. Linner, *Sex and Society in Sweden* (Pantheon, 1967)

B. Malinowski, *The Sexual Life of Savages* (Routledge & Kegan Paul, 1932)

D. Morris, *The Naked Ape* (Cape, 1967)

E. S. Morrison and M. U. Price, *Values in Sexuality* (Hart, 1974)

P. Perry, *Your Guide to the Opposite Sex* (Pitman, 1970)

W. B. Pomeroy, *Boys and Sex* (Delacourt Press, 1968)

W. B. Pomeroy, *Girls and Sex* (Delacourt Press, 1969)

L. C. Schaefer, *Women and Sex* (Hutchinson, 1974)

A. Skolnick, *The Intimate Environment* (Little, Brown & Co., 1974)

L. Tiger and R. Fox, *The Imperial Animal* (Secker & Warburg, 1972)

N. Weisstein, *Kinder, Kücher, Kirche as Scientific Law: Psychology Constructs the Female* (New England Free Press, 1968)

P. Whiting, 'Female Sexuality: its Political Implications' in M. Wandor (ed.) *The Body Politic* (Stage 1 Books, 1978)

Fiction

A. Christie, *Sparkling Cyanide* (Collins, 1945)

M. French, *The Women's Room* (André Deutsch, 1978)

L. P. Hartley, *The Go-Between* (Hamish Hamilton, 1953)

U. le Guin, *The Left Hand of Darkness* (Macdonald, 1969)

C. McCullers, *The Member of the Wedding* (Barrie & Jenkins, 1972)

V. Nabokov, *Lolita* (Weidenfeld & Nicholson, 1959)